PEDIATRIC
Drug Doses

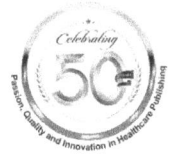

PEDIATRIC Drug Doses

Fourth Edition

GL Chattri MBBS MD MHA
Consultant Pediatrician and Neonatologist
Mahakoshal Hospital
Seth Mannulal Jagannathdas Trust Hospital and
Research Centre
and
Metro Hospital
Jabalpur, Madhya Pradesh, India

Foreword
Avyakt Agarwal

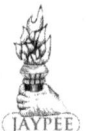

JAYPEE BROTHERS MEDICAL PUBLISHERS
The Health Sciences Publisher
New Delhi | London

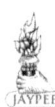
Jaypee Brothers Medical Publishers (P) Ltd.

Headquarters
Jaypee Brothers Medical Publishers (P) Ltd
EMCA House
23/23-B, Ansari Road, Daryaganj
New Delhi - 110 002, India
Landline: +91-11-23272143, +91-11-23272703
+91-11-23282021, +91-11-23245672
Email: jaypee@jaypeebrothers.com

Corporate Office
Jaypee Brothers Medical Publishers (P) Ltd
4838/24, Ansari Road, Daryaganj
New Delhi 110 002, India
Phone: +91-11-43574357
Fax: +91-11-43574314
Email: jaypee@jaypeebrothers.com

Overseas Office
J.P. Medical Ltd
83 Victoria Street, London
SW1H 0HW (UK)
Phone: +44 20 3170 8910
Fax: +44 (0)20 3008 6180
Email: info@jpmedpub.com

Website: www.jaypeebrothers.com
Website: www.jaypeedigital.com

© 2021, Jaypee Brothers Medical Publishers

The views and opinions expressed in this book are solely those of the original contributor(s)/author(s) and do not necessarily represent those of editor(s) of the book.

All rights reserved. No part of this publication may be reproduced, stored or transmitted in any form or by any means, electronic, mechanical, photocopying, recording or otherwise, without the prior permission in writing of the publishers.

All brand names and product names used in this book are trade names, service marks, trademarks or registered trademarks of their respective owners. The publisher is not associated with any product or vendor mentioned in this book.

Medical knowledge and practice change constantly. This book is designed to provide accurate, authoritative information about the subject matter in question. However, readers are advised to check the most current information available on procedures included and check information from the manufacturer of each product to be administered, to verify the recommended dose, formula, method and duration of administration, adverse effects and contraindications. It is the responsibility of the practitioner to take all appropriate safety precautions. Neither the publisher nor the author(s)/editor(s) assume any liability for any injury and/or damage to persons or property arising from or related to use of material in this book.

This book is sold on the understanding that the publisher is not engaged in providing professional medical services. If such advice or services are required, the services of a competent medical professional should be sought.

Every effort has been made where necessary to contact holders of copyright to obtain permission to reproduce copyright material. If any have been inadvertently overlooked, the publisher will be pleased to make the necessary arrangements at the first opportunity. The **CD/DVD-ROM** (if any) provided in the sealed envelope with this book is complimentary and free of cost. **Not meant for sale**.

Inquiries for bulk sales may be solicited at: jaypee@jaypeebrothers.com

Pediatric Drug Doses
First Edition: 2010
Second Edition: 2012
Third Edition: 2016
Fourth Edition: **2021**
ISBN: 978-93-90281-31-2

Dedicated to
*Late (Professor) Dr Rajpoot VJ Sir (Indore),
who taught me the art of pediatrics*

Foreword

One of the areas of deficiency is the lack of easily available information on pediatric drug dosing for front line caregivers. Ideally, all persons involved in the treatment of critically ill infants and children should have the basic knowledge about pediatric drug dosing along with the basic clinical skills. This handbook is a good attempt to do just that. It is a concise and useful guide on all the aspects of care related to pediatric drug dosing.

The information and lessons presented in this book will help those who care for the critically ill child; if studied and kept close at hand, it would bolster their confidence and lessen their anxiety related to drug information (indications, doses, brand names, etc.).

This book is a welcome addition to the pediatric literature. It is a reasonable compromise between voluminous and complex textbooks.

Avyakt Agarwal MD
Assistant Professor
Department of Pediatrics
Netaji Subhash Chandra Bose Medical College
Jabalpur, Madhya Pradesh, India

Preface to the Fourth Edition

Welcome to this edition of the *Pediatric Drug Doses*. Tradition of this publication began in 2010. I am very thankful to all who accepted and appreciated its previous editions. I am satisfied that my efforts have served the felt need of the readers. I have tried to retain the format of previous edition to avoid new feeling and shall continue to enjoy the same patronage of the reading in this edition. This book is not meant to be an alternative to time-tested exhaustive textbooks on drug doses, but meant to be a concise companion for all health professionals dealing with pediatric population on day-to-day basis because it is humanly not possible to remember the wide range of medications currently used in pediatrics. The drugs for malignant disorders have been not included due to variety of protocols followed individually. Drugs of which safety and efficacy in children is not established are not added.

In this edition, existing drugs are updated and expanded, a few drugs are omitted, and many more drugs and useful tables are added. In this edition, the advice of several readers and their suggestions have been incorporated. Although every possible effort is made to ensure the accuracy, reliability, errors and omissions of material presented in this book, the ultimate responsibility rests with the prescribing person because some errors may remain.

GL Chattri

Preface to the First Edition

I am pleased to have the opportunity to write this first edition of *Pediatric Drug Doses*. It is not intended to compete with the already well-established books. This book is designed to be a practical and convenient guide to the dosing and usage of medications in children.

Pediatric doses vary with the age, weight, surface area and disease, etc. Over dosing may lead to side effects and under dosing will lead to unsatisfactory response or development of resistance in cases of antibiotics.

I did not confine myself to doses only, but extended to provide indication, which is a must before knowing doses, and also included the information such as size of feeding tubes, Foley catheters, endotracheal tubes, laryngoscope blades, oxygen mask according to age and weight; approximate weight and surface area charts; fluid resuscitation formula for burn patients, so that residents do not have to consult too many books while dealing with patients bedside. The aim is to improve the practical utility of the book.

I have made all efforts to check for any mistakes in the text and drug doses, but nobody can be perfect. If you are in any doubt about a treatment or drug doses, always check with another formulary. Due to constant research, it is advised to consult package insert especially for infrequently used drugs and drugs with narrow therapeutic index.

I have written this book for pediatric house officers and registrars particularly keeping in mind, but it will also be useful for consultant pediatricians and general practitioners.

GL Chattri

Acknowledgments

First of all, I would like to thanks all my patients and their families who continue to aid us in our development as pediatricians and in the enrichment of our lives.

I thank to my wife Rashmi, my best friend, for her support and encouragement which made my dream true and my kids, Dhruv and Shlok, who spared me from their share of valuable time in writing this book.

I also thank to Mr Sanjeev Pandey, my friend for his selfless personal and professional support, which have made all this possible.

I sincerely thank Shri Jitendar P Vij (Group Chairman), Mr Ankit Vij (Managing Director), Mr MS Mani (Group President), Dr Madhu Choudhary (Publishing Head–Education), Ms Pooja Bhandari (Production Head), Ms Sunita Katla (Executive Assistant to Group Chairman and Publishing Manager), Ms Samina Khan (Executive Assistant to Director–Content Strategy), Ms Seema Dogra (Cover Visualizer), Mr Rajesh Sharma (Production Coordinator), Mr Laxmidhar Padhiary (Proofreader), and Mr Kapil Dev Sharma (Typesetter) of M/s Jaypee Brothers Medical Publishers (P) Ltd, New Delhi, for publishing this book.

Last but not the least, I would like to thank Dr Sharad Thora, Dr Hemant Jain, and Dr Sameer Agarwal for their guidance and support.

Structure of the Book

All the drugs are listed in their respective group and are covered in short to make the book user-friendly. Drug information is presented in a consistent form at and provides the following:

Generic Name: Indian adopted name.

Uses: Information pertaining to appropriate indications or uses of the drug.

Doses: The amount of drug to be typically given or taken during therapy in general and in certain specific conditions. For selected drugs, the dosing adjustment in renal and/or hepatic impairment should be made accordingly.

Brands: Common trade names available in India.

Combinations: If any.

So, if one has reached to the final or probable diagnosis, then this book will provide the remaining information—drugs which can be prescribed, dosages, brands and forms available, and mode of administration.

Contents

1. Analgesics — 1
2. Antiasthmatics — 11
3. Antiarrhythmics — 17
4. Antibiotics — 21
5. Anticoagulants — 54
6. Antidepressants — 56
7. Antidotes/Poisoning — 59
8. Antiemetics — 65
9. Antiepileptics — 69
10. Antifungals — 80
11. Antigout Agents — 86
12. Anthelmintics — 88
13. Antihistamines — 92
14. Antihypertensives — 97
15. Antileprotics — 105
16. Antimalarials — 107
17. Antimyasthenics — 113
18. Antiprotozoals — 115
19. Anxiolytics/Sedatives/Antipsychotics — 118
20. Antiretrovirals — 122
21. Antitubercular — 126
22. Antispasmodics — 131
23. Antitoxins — 133
24. Antiulcers/Antisecretory — 135
25. Antivirals — 137
26. Cardiac Shocks and Failures — 143
27. Chelating Agents — 145
28. Colony-stimulating Factors — 147
29. Corticosteroids — 150
30. Diuretics — 155

31.	Drugs Used for Controlling Bleeding	159
32.	Supplements and Fluid Replacements	161
33.	H$_2$ Antagonists	164
34.	Immunoglobulins	165
35.	Laxatives/Stool Softeners	169
36.	Minerals	172
37.	Nutritional Supplements	174
38.	Pituitary Hormones	176
39.	Plasma Volume Expanders	178
40.	Scabicidal Agents	180
41.	Skeletal Muscle Relaxants	182
42.	Skin/Acne Drugs	185
43.	Sympathomimetics	187
44.	Thyroid and Antithyroid Agents	190
45.	Vaccines	192
46.	Vasodilators	199
47.	Vitamins	200

Miscellaneous Drugs	206
Appendices	221

Appendix 1: Tables 221
Appendix 2: Administering Medicines to Children 233
Appendix 3: General Instructions on Immunization 234
Appendix 4: Age-based Formula for Selecting Endotracheal Tube Size 235

Index	237

Symbols and Abbreviations

ACE	Angiotensin-converting Enzyme
ACTH	Adrenocorticotropic Hormone
ADHD	Attention Deficit Hyperactivity Disorder
ADS	Antidiphtheric Serum
AEDS	Antiepileptic Drugs
AIDS	Acquired Immunodeficiency Syndrome
ANC	Absolute Neutrophil Count
AOM	Acute Otitis Media
APTT	Activated Partial Thromboplastin Time
ARF	Acute Renal Failure
ASD	Autism Spectrum Disorder
AV	Atrioventricular Block
BA	Bronchial Asthma
BCG	Bacillus Calmette-Guérin
BD	Twice a Day
BP	Blood Pressure
BPD	Bronchopulmonary Dysplasia
BSA	Body Surface Area
CAH	Congenital Adrenal Hyperplasia
CCID	Cell Culture Infective Dose
CHD	Congenital Heart Disease
CHF	Congestive Heart Failure
CLD	Chronic Lung Disease
CMV	Cytomegalovirus
CNS	Central Nervous System
CP	Cerebral Palsy
CPM	Chlorpheniramine
CSF	Cerebrospinal Fluid
CSOM	Chronic Suppurative Otitis Media
DCL	Diffuse Cutaneous Leishmaniasis

DEC	Diethyl Carbamazine
DIC	Disseminated Intravascular Coagulation
DM	Diabetes Mellitus
DPT	Diphtheria, Pertussis and Tetanus
E/E	Eye/Ear
ECG	Electrocardiograph
ELISA	Enzyme-linked Immunosorbent Assay
ENT	Ear, Nose, and Throat
EPO	Erythropoietin
ET	Endotracheal Tube
G6PD	Glucose-6-Phosphate Dehydrogenase
GBHC	Gamma Benzene Hexachloride
GERD	Gastroesophageal Reflux Disease
g	Gram
GI	Gastrointestinal
HA	Headache
HBsAG	Surface Antigen of the Hepatitis B Virus
HDN	Hemolytic Disease of the Newborn
h	Hour
HIV	Human Immunodeficiency Virus
hs	At Bedtime
HSV	Herpes Simplex Virus
HT	Hypertension
HZV	Herpes Zoster Virus
ICP	Intracranial Pressure
ICT	Intracranial Tension
Id	Intradermal
Ig	Immunoglobulin
IM	Intramuscular
IPV	Inactivated Polio Vaccine
ITP	Idiopathic Thrombocytopenic Purpura
IVH	Intraventricular Hemorrhage
IVIG	Intravenous Immunoglobulin
IV	Intravenous
IVP	Intravenous Push

JRA	Juvenile Rheumatoid Arthritis
kg	Kilogram
LAB	Lactic Acid Bacillus
LBW	Low Birth Weight
LCL	Localized Cutaneous Leishmaniasis
LFT	Liver FunctionTest
LMWH	Low Molecular Weight Heparin
LRTI	Lower Respiratory Tract Infection
MDI	Metered-doseInhaler
mg	Milligram
Min	Minute
mL	Milliliter
ML	Mucosal Leishmaniasis
MMR	Measles, Mumps and Rubella
MRSA	Methicillin-Resistant *Staphylococcus aureus*
N/V	Nausea/Vomiting
NB	Newborn
NEC	Necrotizing Enterocolitis
Ng	Nasogastric
NSAID	Nonsteroidal Anti-inflammatory Drug
NS	Normal Saline
od	Once a Day
OM	Otitis Media
OPV	Oral Polio Vaccine
PBP	Plasma Binding Protiens
PCM	Paracetamol
PDA	Patent Ductus Arteriosus
PFU	Plaque-forming Unit
PM	Pyrimethamine
PNA	Postnatal Age
PO	Per Oral
PR	Per Rectum
PRP	Polyribosylribitolphosphate
PSVT	Paroxysmal Supraventricular Tachycardia
PT	Prothrombin Time

qid	Four Times Per Day
RDA	Recommended Daily Allowance
RDS	Respiratory Distress Syndrome
rHuEPO	Recombinant Human Erythropoietin
RSV	Respiratory Syncytial Virus
RT	Respiratory Tract
RTI	Respiratory Tract Infection
SC	Subcutaneous
SD	Sulfadoxine
SGPT	Serum Glutamic-pyruvic Transaminase
SJS	Steven's Jhonson Syndrome
SLE	Systemic Lupus Erythematosus
SL	Sublingual
SMZ	Sulfamethoxazole
SSTI	Skin and Soft Tissue Infection
TB	Tuberculosis
tds	Thrice a Day
tid	Three Times a Day
TIG	Tetanus Immunoglobulin
TLC	Total Lung Capacity
TMP	Trimethoprim
TPN	Total Parenteral Nutrition
TT	Tetanus Toxoid
UMN	Upper Motor Neuron
URTI	Upper Respiratory Tract Infection
UTI	Urinary Tract Infection
VL	Visceral Leishmaniasis
VZIG	Varicella Zoster Immunoglobulin
VZV	Varicella Zoster Virus
WBC	White Blood Cell
μg	Microgram
<	Less than
≤	Less than or Equal to
>	Greater than
≥	Greater than or Equal to

Analgesics

chapter 1

NON-NARCOTIC ANALGESIC

These are used to control mild to moderate pain, fever and various inflammatory conditions. Most nonopioid analgesics inhibit prostaglandin synthesis peripherally for analgesic effect and centrally for antipyretic effect. Use cautiously in patients with a history of bleeding disorders, gastrointestinal (GI) bleeding, and severe hepatic, renal or cardiovascular (CV) disease. Administer salicylates and nonsteroidal anti-inflammatory drugs (NSAIDs) after meals or with food or an antacid to minimize gastric irritation. Patients on long-term therapy of aspirin, salicylates and NSAIDs may need to be withheld prior to surgery.

ACETYLSALICYLIC ACID

Uses: Treatment of inflammation, fever, and mild to moderate pain.

Dosage: PO
- Pain and fever: 10–15 mg/kg/dose q 4-6 hr
- Anti-inflammatory: 60–90 mg/kg/day in divided doses
- Antiplatelet effect: 3–10 mg/kg/day, single daily dose
- Kawasaki disease: 80–100 mg/kg/day divided q 6 hr
- Rheumatic fever: 60–100 mg/kg/day divided q 6 hr

Brands: Ecosprin tablet—75, 150 and 325 mg. Delisprin tablet—75 and 150 mg. Zosprin tablet—100 and 150 mg.
- Contraindicated in chickenpox or if there is flu-like symptom, hepatic failure, bleeding disorder, erosive gastritis, peptic ulcer, bronchial asthma. Discontinue the drug if hearing loss or tinnitus occurs.

AURANOFIN

Uses: Management of active stage of classic or definite rheumatoid, psoriatic arthritis.

Dosage: PO
- Starting: 0.1 mg/kg/day in two divided doses
- Maintenance: 0.15 mg/kg/day (maximum: 0.2 mg/kg/day)

Brands: Capsule; Ridaura 3 mg; tablet; Goldar 3 mg.
- Contraindicated in blood dyscrasias, congestive heart failure (CHF), necrotizing enterocolitis (NEC), systemic lupus erythematosus (SLE), leukopenia, urticaria, etc. Stop therapy if platelet count <100,000/mm^3, white blood count (WBC) <4,000/mm^3.

CELECOXIB

Uses: Osteoarthritis, rheumatoid arthritis, juvenile rheumatoid arthritis (JRA), ankylosing spondylitis.

Dosage: PO—> 2years: 10-25 kg; 50 mg twice daily. >25 kg; 100 mg twice daily.

Brands: 100, 200 mg cap; Celcib, Celib, Calcibra.

DICLOFENAC SODIUM

Uses: Mild to moderate pain, juvenile rheumatoid arthritis (JRA).

Dosage: PO: 2–3 mg/kg/day divided q 4 hr.

Brands: 50 and 100 mg tablet; Agile MR, Diclofam, Diclomax.
- Also available in topical formulation as gel; Diclonac, Nac, Voveran 1% gel; transdermal patch, Nupatch. Contraindicated in GI bleeding, ulcer disease, aspirin triad. Use with caution in hypertension, bronchial asthma, CHF, fluid retention, dehydration, etc.

ETODOLAC

Uses: Osteoarthritis, rheumatoid arthritis, pain.

Dosage: PO: 0-20 mg/kg/day in 3 divided doses (maximum: 100 mg/day).

Brands: 400 mg tablet; Etogesic, Etura.

ETORICOXIB

Uses: Osteoarthritis, rheumatoid arthritis, ankylosing spondylitis, acute gout.

Dosage: PO—>16-18 years age, orally—osteroarthritis—30 mg once only. Rheumatoid and ankylosing spondylitis—90 mg once daily. Acute gout—120 mg once daily for 8 days.

Brands: 60, 90, 120 mg tablet; Etrobox, Etorax.

IBUPROFEN

Uses: Fever, pain, JRA, Cystic fibrosis, Patent ductus arteriosus (PDA), migraine.

Dosage: PO
- Fever, pain: 4–10 mg/kg/dose q 6–8 hr (maximum: 40 mg/kg/day)
- JRA: 30–50 mg/kg/day in four divided doses (maximum: 2.4 g/day)
- Cystic fibrosis: 20–30 mg/kg twice daily for 4 years
- PDA: IV—initial dose of 10 mg/kg, followed at 24 hours intervals by two doses of 5 mg/kg
- Migraine: 7.5–10 mg/kg/dose.

Brands: 100 mg/5 mL suspension; Bren, Ibugesic, Febrilix. 200 mg and 400 mg tablet; Brufen, Emflam, Ibugesic, Ibugin.

Combinations: Ibuprofen + Paracetamol:
- 400 mg + 325 mg tablet—Anaflam, Combiflam, Ibucin, Zupar
- 100 mg + 125/5 mL suspension—Anaflam, Zupar
- 100 mg + 162.5 mg/5 mL suspension—Combiflam, Ibucin

Contraindicated in GI bleeding, ulcer disease, aspirin triad. Use with caution in CHF CHF, HT, dehydration, hepatic, and renal patients.

INDOMETHACIN

Uses: PDA closure in neonates, rheumatoid arthritis, nephrogenic diabetes insipidus.

Dosage:
- Neonates (PDA): IV; 0.2 mg/kg initially followed by two doses at 12–24 hours intervals

- Rheumatoid/inflammatory disorders: PO: 1–2 mg/kg/day in 2–4 doses (maximum: 4 mg/kg/day)
- Nephrogenic diabetes insipidus: PO—2 mg/kg/day (for patients having inadequate response to diuretics alone may benefit from its addition).

Brands: 25 and 50 mg capsule; Artisid, Indocap, Microcid, etc.
- Contraindicated in premature neonates with NEC, impaired renal functions, intraventricular hemorrhage (IVH), bleeding, thrombocytopenia. It may decrease the antihypertensive effect of diuretics. Hold enteral feeds for 12 hours after last dose.

KETOROLAC

Uses: Treatment of ocular itch associated with seasonal allergic conjunctivitis.

Dosage: Children >3 years: 1 drop in eyes 4 times/day; up to 7 days.

Brands: 0.5% drop; Acular, Doloket, Ketanov, Ketodrop, etc.

Administration: Apply pressure over lacrimal sac for 2 minute after application to avoid absorption and systemic effects.

MEFENAMIC ACID

Uses: Fever, pain, rheumatoid disorders.

Dosage: PO—should not be given for >7 days.
- Fever: 3 mg/kg/dose upto 3 times per day.
- Rheumatoid disorder: 10–25 mg/kg/day q 6 hr.

Brands: 100, 250 and 500 mg tablet; 100 and 50 mg/5 mL suspension; Meftal, Ponstan.

Combinations:
- Mefenamic + Paracetamol: 500 + 450 mg tablet; MeftalForte.
- Mefenamic + Dicyclomine: 250 + 10 mg tablet; Meftalspas.

MELOXICAM

Uses: Pain, rheumatoid arthritis, juvenile idiopathic arthritis, musculoskeletal pain.

Dosage: PO: 12-18 years <50 kg, 7.5 mg; >50 kg 15 mg once daily. In renal failure maximum dose 7.5 mg once daily.

Brands: 15 mg tablet; M-Cam, Melflam.

NAPROXEN

Uses: Fever, pain, inflammation and rheumatoid disorders.

Dosage: PO—for children >2 years of age:
- Pain: 5–7 mg/kg/dose q 8-12 hr
- JRA/inflammatory disease: 10–15 mg/kg/day in two divided doses (maximum: 1,000 mg/day).

Brands: 250 mg tablet; Artagen, Nalyxan, Naprosyn.

NIMESULIDE

Uses: Pain, myalgia, arthritis, thrombophlebitis, dental pain, postoperative, sinusitis, sports injury.

Dosage: PO—children >12 years 5 mg/kg/day in 2-3 divided doses.

Brands: 50 mg/5 mL susp; 100 mg tab; Nimulid, Nimegesic.

PARACETAMOL/ACETAMINOPHEN

Uses: Mild to moderate pain and fever; migraine. Do not have an anti-inflammatory or antirheumatic effect.

Dosage:
- Neonates: PO—rectal; 10–15 mg/kg/dose q 6-8 hr
- Infants and children: PO—10–15 mg/kg/dose q 4-6 hr
- Rectal: 10–20 mg/kg/dose q 4-6 hr
- IM: 5 mg/kg/dose.

Brands: 150 mg/mL drops; 120 mg/5 mL syrup; 500 and 650 mg tablet; Calpol, Lanol. 80 and 170 mg suppository; Anamol, Junimol. 150 mg/mL injection; Fevastin, Febrinil, Mol.
- Overdoses of paracetamol can be treated with acetylcysteine.

PIROXICAM

Uses: Rheumatoid and inflammatory disorders.

Dosage: PO—0.2–0.3 mg/kg/day as single dose (maximum: 15 mg/kg/day).

Brands: 10 and 20 mg tablet and capsule; Brexic, Minicam, Paricam. Use with caution in infants and children.

TOLMETIN

Uses: Inflammatory and rheumatoid disorders (JRA).

Dosage: Children >2 years of age: PO
- Anti-inflammatory: 15–20 mg/kg/day in 3–4 divided doses (maximum: 30 mg/kg/day)
- Analgesic: 5–7 mg/kg/dose q 6–8 hr

Brands: 200 mg tablet; 400 mg capsule; Tolectin.

NARCOTIC ANALGESIC

Used for management of moderate to severe pain. Fentanyl is also used as a general anesthetic adjunct. Opioids binds to receptors in the central nervous system (CNS), where they acts as a agonists of endogenously occurring opioid peptides (eukephlins and endorphins). The result is alteration to the perception of and response to pain. Use cautiously in patients with undiagnosed abdominal pain, head trauma, liver disease. Use smaller doses in elderly and those with respiratory disease.

CODEINE

Uses: Mild-to-moderate pain; for nonproductive cough use in lower doses.

Dosage:
- Pain: 0.5-1 mg/kg/dose q 4-6 hr (maximum: 60 mg/dose)
- Cough: 1-1.5 mg/kg/day divided q 4-6 hr (not recommended in children <2 years of age).

Brands: Codeine linctus; Codeine sulfate 15 mg + menthol, 0.2 mg/5 mL. Phensedyl, Codokuff; Codeine phosphate 10 mg + Chlorpheniramine 4 mg/5 mL. Lincotuss; Codeine phosphate 15 mg/5 mL.

- Increase fluid and fiber intake to avoid constipation
- Contraindicated in pre-existing respiratory illness, asthma, and raised intracranial pressure (ICP). It can causes constipation, nausea, anorexia, vomiting, sedation, dizziness.

FENTANYL

Uses: Sedation, pain relief, preoperative medication, adjunct to anesthesia.

Dosage:
- Neonates and infants: IV– intermittent dose are 1–4 µg/kg/dose; may be repeated q 2-4 hr; continuous infusion: 0.5–5 µg/kg/h
- Older infants and children (1–12 year) Pain; IM, IV: 1–3 µg/kg/dose; may be repeated after 30 minutes; continuous infusion: 1–5 µg/kg/h
- Children >12 years; Pain: IM, IV: 0.5–1 µg/kg/dose; may be repeated after ½ to 1 hour
- Anesthesia: IM, IV: 2–50 µg/kg.

Brands: 50 µg/mL injection; Fendrop, Fenilate, Fent, Trofentyl. Patch of 25, 50 and 100 µg/h, Duragesic.

Administration: For IV administer slowly over 5–10 minutes. Rapid IV infusion may cause skeletal muscle rigidity, impaired ventilation, apnea, laryngospasm.
- Contraindicated in raised ICP, severe respiratory depression, hepatic or renal problems. Physical and psychological dependence may occurs with prolonge use.

MORPHINE SULFATE

Uses: Pain relief; relieves dyspnea of left ventricular failure and pulmonary edema; preanesthetic medication.

Dosage:
- Neonates: IV, IM, SC—continuous infusion: 0.01-0.03 mg/kg/h; intermittent dose: 0.05-0.1 mg/kg/dose q 2-4 hr
- Infants and children: IV, IM, SC—0.1–0.2 mg/kg/dose q 2–4h (maximum: 15 mg/dose). PO—0.2–0.5 mg/kg/ dose q 4-6 hr
- >12 years: 3–4 mg; may be repeated after 5 minutes as required.

Brands: 10 and 30 mg tablet; Duramor, Morcontin. 10 mg/mL injection; morphine sulfate.

Administration: Administer IV over 15–30 minutes at a final concentration of 0.5-5 mg/mL

- Contraindicated in respiratory depression, GI obstruction, acute or severe asthma, liver or renal problems. Neonates and infants <3 months are more susceptible to respiratory depression.

PENTAZOCINE

Uses: Relief of moderate to severe pain, sedative prior to surgery.

Dosage: Efficacy and safety not confirmed below 12 years. Children >12 years: PO—50 mg/dose q 3-4 hr; (maximum: 600 mg/day). IV or IM dose is 1/3rd of PO dose.

Brands: 25 mg tablet; Fortwin. 30 mg/mL injection; Fortwin, Pentawin, Susevin.

PETHIDINE/MEPERIDINE

Uses: Pain, adjunct to anesthesia, and preoperative sedation.

Dosage: IV, IM: 1–1.5 mg/kg/dose q 3-4 hr as needed; 1–2 mg/kg as preoperative medication single dose (maximum: 100 mg/dose).

Brands: 50 mg/mL injection; Pethidine hydrochloride.

Administration: For IV, dilute to 1–10 mg/mL and to be given over 15–30 minutes.

- Use with caution in head injury, raised ICP and in young children. Pethidine though used in combination with chlorpromazine and promethazine in lytic cocktail; this mixture may have a higher rate of adverse effects compared to alternative sedatives and analgesics.

TRAMADOL HYDROCHLORIDE

Uses: Management of moderate to severe pain.

Dosage: PO/IV—children >14 years, 0.5-1 mg/kg q 8 hourly.

Brands: 50 mg tab; 100 mg injection; Anatram, Dolfi, Nobligan.

TOPICAL ANALGESIC

BENZOCAINE

Uses: Toothache, sore throat pain, hemorrhoids, rectal fissures, minor burns, etc.

Dosage: Apply to affected area as needed. Mouth/throat, usage should not exceed 2 days.

Brand: 7.5% gel; T-JEL.

LIDOCAINE

Uses: Local anesthetic, relief of pain in postherpetic neuralgia, ventricular arrhythmias.

Dosage:
- Topical: Apply as needed but maximum dose is 3 mg/kg/dose; do not repeat within 2 hours
- Injectable local anesthetic: As needed but maximum dose is 4.5 mg/kg/dose; do not repeat within 2 hours
- Arrhythmias: Loading dose 1 mg/kg; continuous infusion 20–50 μg/kg/min (20 μg/kg/min in patients with shock, mild CHF, liver disease, cardiac arrest)
- Postherpetic neuralgia: Apply patch to affected areas (maximum: 3 patch).

Brands: Gesicain, Lignox: 5% injection; 2% jelly, 5% ointment, 4% topical solution. Xylocaine: 1%, 2% and 5% injection; 2% jelly, 5% ointment, spray, 4% topicalsolution, 2% viscous. Xylocard: 50 mL vial (1 mL = 21.3 mg), shield ointment.

Combinations: Shield ointment contains lidocaine 3%, Hydrocortisone acetate 0.25%, zinc oxide 5%, allantoin 0.5%.

Administration: For IV, dilution should be 8–20 mg/mL. Lidocaine solutions containing epinephrine should not be used for treatment of arrhythmias and preservative containing solutions should not be used for IV.

URINARY ANALGESIC

PHENAZOPYRIDINE

Uses: Symptomatic relief of urinary burning, frequency and urgency associated with UTI or urologic procedures.

Dosage: PO—12 mg/kg/day divided q 8 hr

Brands: Pyridium 200 mg tablet

Combinations: Phenazopyridine + Nitrofurantoin: 200 + 50 mg tablet; Nephrogesic.

- It is not an antibiotic and do not treat infections. May discoloration of urine to orange or red.

Antiasthmatics

chapter 2

These are drugs used for the treatment of bronchial asthma. They are classified according to their role in asthma management, as either quick relief (e.g., salbutamol, levosalbutamol) or long-term control (prednisolone, beclomethasone) medication.

ADRENALINE/EPINEPHRINE

Refer Chapter 43 Sympathomimetic's.

AMINOPHYLLINE

Uses: As bronchodilator, apnea of prematurity, increase diaphragmatic contractility.

Dosage:
- Apnea of prematurity: PO—IV; loading dose of 6 mg/kg followed by maintenance dose of 2.5–3 mg/kg/dose q 12 hr. Should be given very slowly.
- Acute bronchospasm: IV; loading dose of 6 mg/kg diluted to 1 mg/mL and infuse over 30 minute followed by 0.5–1 mg/kg/hr as continuous infusion, if already on oral therapy, omit loading dose. PO: 15–20 mg/kg/day divided q 8 hr.

Brands: 100 mg tablet; 25 mg/mL injection; Aminophylline.

- May cause seizures, tachyarrhythmias, feeding intolerance in neonates, gastroesophageal reflux, vomiting, CNS irritability. With hold dose for heart rate >180 beats/min.

BAMBUTEROL

Uses: Long-term therapy of asthma.

Doses: PO—children 2-5 years: 5 mg, 6-12 years: 10 mg. Single dose at bed time.

Brands: 10, 20 mg tablet; 5 mg/mL suspension; Bambudil, Betaday, Roburol.

BECLOMETHASONE

Use: Long-term control of asthma.

Dosage: Inhalation 100–800 µg/day in divided doses depending on severity.

Brands: 50, 100, 200 and 250 µg/actuation; Beclate inhaler. 50, 100, 250 µg/actuation; Becoride inhaler. 100 and 200 µg rotacap; Beclate, Bevent.

Combinations: Beclomethasone + Salbutamol: 50 + 100 µg inhaler. 100 + 400 µg rotacaps; Aerocort, Ventplus.
- To reduce chances of oral candidiasis, rinse mouth after inhalation. Use spacer device for inhalational corticosteroids in children for better lung delivery and less local toxicity.
- Chronic asthma patient require long-term and regular therapy.

BUDESONIDE

Uses: Allergic rhinitis, long-term prophylaxis, and maintenance therapy of asthma.

Dosage: 100–600 µg/day in divided doses depending upon severity. Nasal spray 2 times/day.

Brands: 0.5 and 1 mg/2 mL; Respule Budate, Budecort. 100 and 200 µg/actuation inhaler; Budecort.100 and 200 µg rotacaps; Budecort. 50 µg/dose nasal spray; Pulmicort.
- Use with precautions in patient with pulmonary tuberculosis (TB), systemic infection and ocular herpes.

CICLESONIDE

Uses: Bronchial asthma, allergic rhinitis.

Dosage: Inhaler given by MDI in a dose range of 80–640 µg/ day depending upon the severity of the disease. Nasal spray: 50-200 µg/day in divided doses.

Brands: 80 and 160 µg/spray MDI; Ciclez, Ciclohale, Osonide. 50 µg/puff nasal spray; Ciplospray, Osonase.

DOXOPHYLLINE

Use: Maintenance therapy in patient suffering with asthma.

Dosage: PO—children >2 years; 12-18 mg/kg/day in single or two divided doses (maximum: 200 mg BD). If nocturnal symptoms are more prefer single eveningdose.

Brands: 100 mg/5 mL syrup; 400 mg tablet; Doxoril, Doxovent, Doxobid.
- May cause nausea and vomiting, dyspepsia, palpitation, tremor, insomania.

FLUTICASONE

Use: Chronic asthma.

Dosage: Depends upon severity and systemic corticosteroids use. 100–600 µg/day divided q 12 hr.

Brands: 0.5 mg Respule; 25, 50 and 125 µg/actuation inhaler; 50, 100 and 250 µg rotacaps; Flohale.
- May cause oral candidiasis, change of voice, adrenal suppression, growth retardation, cataracts.

FORMOTEROL

Use: Treatment and prophylaxis of asthma.

Dosage: >5 years of age—12 µg twice daily 12 hours apart.

Brands: 12 µg rotacaps and inhaler; Foratec.

Combination: Formoterol + Budesonide: 6 + 200 and 6 µg + 400 µg rotacaps and inhaler; Foracort, Vent-FB.

IPRATROPIUM

Use: Acute and chronic asthma.

Dosage:
- Neonates: 25 µg/kg/dose 3 times/day as nebulization

- Infants and children: 125–250 µg as nebulization or 1–2 puffs 2–3 times/day.

Brands: 250 µg/mL solution for nebulization; Ipramist, Ipravent. 20 µg/actuation inhaler; 40 µg rotacaps; Ipravent and Ipratop.

- May cause tachycardia, drowsiness, xerostomia, blurred vision.

LEVOSALBUTAMOL

Dosage: For children >4 years of age: Nebulization—0.075 mg/kg for 3 doses q 1-4 hourly (minimum:1.25 mg and maximum: 5 mg). Continuous nebulization: 0.25 mg/kg/hr.

Brands: 1,2 mg tab; 0.5 and 1 mg/5mL susp; 150 µg/puff MDI; Levolin.

MONTELUKAST

Uses: Prophylaxis and chronic treatment of asthma; symptomatic relief of seasonal allergic rhinitis.

Dosage: 1–5 years: 4 mg/day; 6–14 years: 5 mg/day; >14 years: 10 mg/day; given as once evening dose.

Brands: 4, 5 and 10 mg tablet; Emlucast, Montair, Romilast. 4 mg granules; Montair.

- May cause palpitations, headache, elevated liver enzymes, myalgia, fatigue.

SALBUTAMOL

Use: Prevention and relief of bronchospasm in asthma.

Dosage:
- Nebulization: Neonates; 0.1–0.5 mg/kg/dose q 6 hourly. Children; 0.15–2.5 mg/dose q 4–6 hr (minimum: 2.5 mg). Continuous nebulization for severe exacerbation: 0.5 mg/kg/hr.
- Inhaler: 100–800 µg/day in divided dose
- PO—Neonates: 0.1–0.3 mg/kg/dose q 6–8 hr. Children: <6 years: 0.1–0.2 mg/kg/dose TDS, 6–12 years: 2 mg/dose TDS or QID, >12 years: 2–4 mg TDS or QID.

Brands: 2 and 4 mg tablet; 2 mg/5 mL syrup; 100 µg/actuation inhaler; Asthalin, Ventorlin. 2.5 mg/2.5 mL respule; Asthalin, Derihaler. 200 and 400 µg rotacaps; Asthalin.

Combinations: Salbutamol + Beclomethasone: 100 + 50 µg inhaler; Aerocort, Salbair-B. 200 + 100 µg rotacaps; Aerocort.
- May cause tachycardia, palpitation, hyperglycemia, tremor, CNS stimulation, insomnia, flushing.

SALMETEROL

Use: Maintenance treatment of asthma.

Dosage: 25–50 µg twice daily in children >4 years of age.

Brands: 25 µg/actuation inhaler; 50 µg rotacaps; Serobid.

SODIUM CROMOGLYCATE

Uses: Prophylaxis for chronic asthma, allergic rhinitis, vernal keratoconjunctivitis.

Dosage: Nebulization; 20 mg 2–3 times/day. Inhaler; 1–2 puffs 3–4 times/day. Intranasal in >2 years of age, 1 spray 3–4 times/day. Ophthalmic in >4 years of age: 1–2 drop 3–4 times/day.

Brands: 5 mg/actuation inhaler; 20 mg/2 mL respule; 20 mg rotacaps; 2% eye drop; Cromal. 1 mg/actuation; 2% eye drop; Fintal. 2.8 mg/dose nasal spray; Fintal, Cromal AQ.

TERBUTALINE

Use: Bronchodilator in asthma.

Dosage: PO—0.05 mg/kg/dose q 8 hr (maximum: 5 mg). SC: 0.005–0.01 mg/kg/dose; may be repeated in 15–20 minutes for 3 doses (maximum: 0.4 mg/dose). Nebulization: 0.01–0.03mg/kg (minimum:0.1mg). Inhalation: 1–2 puffs q 6–8 hr.

Brands: 2.5 mg tablet; Asmaterb, Bricanyl, Brontaline. 1.5 mg/5 mL syrup; Bricaline, Bricanyl. 0.5 mg/mL injection; Bricanyl, Terbutaline Sulfate. 250 µg/actuation inhaler; 10 mg/mL nebulizing solution; Bricanyl. 5 mL syrup; Dilo-BM, Terbutaline Sulfate 1.25 mg; Ambroxol hydrochloride 30 mg, Guaiphenesin 30 mg, flavored syrup base containing menthol color.
- May cause tachycardia, flushing, headache, tremor, hypokalemia, dry throat.

THEOPHYLLINE

Uses: Treatment of asthma.

Doses: PO—>6 months: 5 mg/kg/dose 3–4 times/day; adjust dose according to response. Sustained release preperations; 8–12 years, 10 mg/kg/dose and 12–18 years, 8 mg/kg/dose (maximum: 500 mg/dose).

Brands: 50 mg/5 mL syrup;Theoped.

- Ideally tablet and syrup should be taken after food.Seizures can be exacerbated in patients taking theophylline preperations.

ZAFIRLUKAST

Use: Maintenance treatment of asthma.

Doses: PO—5–11 years, 10 mg twice daily. >12 years, 20 mg twice daily. Given 1 hour before or 2 hours after meals.

Brands: 10 and 20 mg tablet; Accolate, Zovair

ZILEUTON

Use: Maintenance treatment of asthma.

Dosage: PO—>12 years; 600 mg 4 times/day.

Brands: 600 mg tab; Zyflo.

Antiarrhythmics

chapter 3

These agents are used for the suppression of cardiac arrhythmias. These corrects arrhythmias by a variety of mechanisms; therapeutic goal is decreased symptomatology and increased hemodynamic performances. Choice of agents depends on etiology of arrhythmia. Treatable causes of arrhythmias should be corrected before therapy is initiated (e.g., electrolyte disturbances, drug toxicity, etc).

ADENOSINE

Uses: Treatment of paroxysmal supraventricular tachycardia (PSVT).

Dosage: Neonates and children– initial dose of 0.05 mg/ kg then increase by 0.05 mg/kg q 2 minutes until a PSVT is terminated or a maximum dose of either 0.25/kg or 12 mg is given.

Brands: 3 mg/mL injection; Adinocor, Adenoject.

- Contraindicated in second or third degree AV block, sick sinus syndrome. Use with caution in asthmatics, patient taking Digoxin, Verapamil. Always administer by IV site closest to the heart as administration into lower extremities may result in failure of therapy or requirement of higher doses and follow each bolus by saline flush.

AMIODARONE

Use: Life-threatening ventricular arrhythmias.

Dosage:
- PO— <1 year of age: 600–800 mg/1.73 m^2/day divided q 12 hr; >1 year of age: 10–20 mg/kg/day divided q 12 hr for 10 days, then 5–10 mg/kg/day. Either arrhythmias are controlled or after 1–4 week of treatment doses are reduced to half

- IV: Loading dose of 5 mg/kg over ½–1 hr; may be repeated up to maximum of 15 mg/kg/day.

Brands: 100 and 200 mg tablet; 50 mg/mL injection; Cardarone, Duron, Tachyra.

- For IV use dilute to 1.5 mg/mL in Dextrose 5% solution. May cause proarrhythmia, nightmares, behavioral changes, hyperglycemia, pneumonitis, skin color changes.

ATROPINE SULFATE

Uses: Preanesthetic medication to inhibit salivation and secretions, sinus bradycardia, organophosphate poisoning, refraction testing in children, uveitis.

Dosage:
- Preanesthesia: IV, IM, SC; <5 kg: 0.02 mg/kg/dose ½an hour before then every 4–6 hour as needed. > 5 kg: 0.01–0.02 mg/kg/dose (maximum: 0.4 mg/dose)
- Sinus bradycardia: Neonates and children– IV, intratracheal; 0.02 mg/kg (minimum: 0.1 mg and maximum: 0.5 mg) may be repeated after 5 minutes once
- Organophosphate poisoning: IV, IM: 0.02–0.05 mg/ kg q10–20 minutes until dry flushed skin, tachycardia, mydriasis, fever is observed then q 1–4 hr for at least 24 hours
- Bronchospasm in children: Inhalation; 0.03–0.05 mg/ kg/dose 3–4 times/day (maximum: 2.5 mg/dose).

Brands: 0.6 mg/mL injection; Atropine sulfate, Tropine. 1% drop and ointment; Atro.

- Give IV by rapid IV push as slow injection may result in paradoxical bradycardia. For intratracheal use dilute with saline to 2–5 mL then give positive pressure ventilations. Contraindicated in thyrotoxicosis, tachycardia, obstructive disease of GI tract, obstructive uropathy
- Effective oxygenation and ventilation must precede atropine treatment of bradycardia.

DISOPYRAMIDE

Uses: Treatment of ventricular arrhythmias and atrial tachyarrhythmias.

Dosage: PO– <1 year: 10–30 mg/kg/day divided q 6 hr; 1–4 years: 10–20 mg/kg/day divided q 6 hr; 4–12 years: 10–15 mg/ kg/day divided q 6 hr.

Brands: 100 mg tablet; Regubeat. 100 and 150 mg capsule; Norpace.
- Contraindicated in second and third degree AV block, cardiogenic shock, avoid along with Erythromycin and Clarithromycin. May cause urinary retention, malaise, constipation, hepatic cholestasis, blurred vision, dizziness.

LIDOCAINE
Refer Topical Analgesic.

MEXILETINE

Uses: Ventricular arrhythmias, congenital myotonia, myotonic dystrophy.

Dosage: PO: 1–4 mg/kg/dose q 8 hr. Start at lower doses and increase according to effect.

Brands: 50 and 150 mg capsule; 25 mg/mL injection; Mexitil.
- Contraindicated in second or third degree block. May cause bradycardia, hypotension, paresthesias, blurred vision, tinnitus, convulsions.

PHENYTOIN
Refer Chapter 9 Antiepileptics.

PROCAINAMIDE

Uses: Ventricular tachycardia, premature ventricular contractions, atrial fibrillation, and paroxysmal atrial tachycardia.

Dosage:
- PO: 15–50 mg/kg/day divided q 3–6 hr (maximum: 4 g/day).
- IV: Loading dose of 3–6 mg/kg/dose to be given over 5 minutes (maximum:100 mg/dose); may be repeated q 5–10 min as needed to maximum of 15 mg/kg. Maintenance dose is 20–80 µg/kg/min (maximum: 2 g/day).

Brands: 250 mg tablet; 100 mg/mL injection; Pronestyl.
- May cause hypotension, arrhythmias, agranulocytosis, neutropenia, hepatomegaly, lupus-like syndrome.

PROPAFENONE HYDROCHLORIDE

Uses: Supraventricular tachyarrhythmias, ventricular tachyarrhythmias, junctional ectopic tachycardia.

Dosage: PO: 10–20 m/kg/day in 2 divided doses; start at lower dose.

IV: 0.2 mg/kg slowly over 10 minutes; can be repeated every 15 minutes up to maximum of 2 mg/kg.

IV infusion: 4 µg/kg/min (under ECG monitoring).

Brands: 10 mg tab; Rhythmonorm.
- Oral tablet should be swallowed as a whole, if crushed the tablet may have a local anesthetic effect.

PROPRANOLOL

Refer Chapter 14 'antihypertensives'.

QUINIDINE SULFATE

Uses: Supraventricular tachycardia, paroxysmal ventricular tachycardia, ventricular ectopics.

Dosage: Test dose is given in 2 mg/kg followed by dose of 30 mg/kg/day divided q 6 hr. Test dose is given for idiosyncratic reaction, intolerance, syncope, thrombocytopenia.

Brands: 100 mg tab; Natcardine. 200 mg tab; Quinidine. 80 mg/mL injection; Quinidine.
- May cause hypotension, heart block, bone marrow suppression, thrombocytopenia.

SOTALOL

Use: Supraventricular and ventricular arrhythmias.

Dosage: 2–8 mg/kg/day divided q8–12 hr.

Brands: 40 and 80 mg tablet; Sotagard.

Antibiotics

chapter 4

Antibiotics are used for treatment and prophylaxis of various bacterial infections.These agents either kill (bactericidal) or inhibit the growth (bacteriostatic) of susceptible pathogenic bacteria.Subdivided into categories depending on chemical similarities and antimicrobial spectrum. Prolonged and inappropriate use of broad spectrum antibiotics may lead to superinfection with fungi or resistant bacteria.Obtain specimens for culture and sensitivity prior to initiating therapy.

Always adopt a rational antibiotic use policy which means use antimicrobials only when indicated and chosing the right agent in the right dose through the right route for right duration.

AMINOGLYCOSIDES

These are a group of antibiotics which are bactericidal against gram-negative bacilli. Acts by inhibiting protein synthesis in bacteria at level of 30S ribosome.

Dosage adjustment in renal impairment is required. Administer other antibiotics, such as penicillins and cephalosporins at least 1 hour before or after giving aminoglycosides,because former inactivates later. May cause ototoxicity, nephrotoxicity, and neuromuscular blockade..

Few indications for serum concentration monitoring include:

- Treatment duration >5 days
- Patients with impaired renal functions
- Infants <3 months of age
- Signs of nephrotoxicity and ototoxicity
- Use of other nephrotoxic agents.
- Clinical need for higher doses or longer intervals.
- Patients on hemodialysis.

Risk factors predisposing to aminoglycosides nephrotoxicity are:
- More the age more the risk
- Pre-existing renal disease
- Use of diuretics
- Effective circulating volume depletion
- Use of other nephrotoxic medications
- Radiographic contrast exposure.

AMIKACIN

Uses: Active against gram –negative bacilli, especially *E.coli, Klebsiella, Proteus, Enterobacter, Serratia, Pseudomonas, Mycobacterium tuberculosis* and *Atypical mycobacteria.*

Dosage: IV/IM neonates:
- PNA <7 days: 1,200–2,000 g; 7.5 mg/kg q 18–24 hr; >2,000 g; 10 mg/kg q 12 hr
- PNA >7 day: 1,200–2,000 g; 7.5 mg/kg q 12–18 hr; >2,000 g;10 mg/kg q 12 hr
- Infants and children: 15–20 mg/kg/day divided, q 8–12 hr
- Antitubercular dose: 15–30 mg/kg/day (maximum dose: 1 g).

Brands: 100, 250, 500 mg/2 mL vial; Amicin, Amikef, Amitex, etc.

Administration: Administer IV slowly over 30–60 minutes; dilution should be 10 mg/mL.

FRAMYCETIN

Uses: Active against many gram negative bacteria (except *Pseudomonas*) and many strains of *Staphylococcus*.Used topically for treatment of skin,eye and ear infection.

Dosage:
- Eye drops: Instill 1-2 drops 3-4 times daily.
- Ointment: Apply about ½ inch to affected area.

Brands: Eye drop and eye ointment 0.5% ; Soframycin eye ointment. 1% ointment; Soframycin skin ointment.

GENTAMICIN SULFATE

Uses: Active against gram-negative bacilli, especially *E. coli, Klebsiella, Proteus, Enterobacter, Serratia, Pseudomonas* and gram-positive *Staphylococcus*.

Dosage: IV/IM:
- Neonates:
  - PNA <7 days: 1,200–2,000 g: 2.5 mg/kg q 12–18 hr; >2,000 g: 2.5 mg/kg q 12 hr
  - PNA >7 days: 1,200–2,000 g: 2.5 mg/kg q 8–12 hr; >2,000 g: 2.5 mg/kg q 8 hr
- Infants and children: 2.5 mg/kg/dose q 8 hr
- Intrathecal: Preservative free preparation for intraventricular or intrathecal use:
  - Neonates: 1 mg/24 hourly
  - Children; 1–2 mg/24 hourly.
- Topical solution: Instill 1–2 drop every 2–4 hourly, upto 2 drops/hour for severe infections.

Brands: 20, 40, 80 mg/vial; Garamycin, Genticyn, Brogaracin, etc. Topical: Genticyn and Garamycin eye/ear drop 0.3%

Administration: Final concentration for IV should not exceed 10 mg/mL.
- Increased otototoxicity with frusomide. Increased neuromuscular blockade, apnea with muscle relaxants.

KANAMYCIN SULFATE

Uses: Active against *Shigella, Klebsiella, E. coli, Serratia, Proteus*, etc. Used as antimycobacterial along with other agents.

Dosage: IV/IM– 15 mg/kg/day divided 12 hourly. Antitubercular; 15–30 mg/kg/day (maximum dose: 1 g).

Brands: 1 g/vial; Kanamycin and Kancin.

NEOMYCIN

Uses: PO before surgery to decrease GI flora and for hyperammonemia to treat diarrhea; used topically for minor skin infections.

Dosage: PO
- Infants: 50 mg/kg/day divided q 6 hr
- Children: 50–100 mg/kg/day divided q 6–8 hr
- Preoperative bowel antisepsis: 90 mg/kg/day divided 4 hourly for 2 days
- Hepatic coma: 2.5–7 g/m^2/day divided every 4–6 hourly for 5–6 days, not to exceed 12 g/day
- Topical: Apply ointment; 1–3 times/day

Brands: 350 mg capsule; Neomycin sulfate.

Causes decrease in absorption of digoxin and bile acids.

NETILMICIN SULFATE

Dosage: IV/IM
- Newborns:
  - <1,200 g, 0–4 weeks: 2.5 mg/kg q 18–24 hr
  - 1,200–2,000 g, 0–7 days: 2.5 mg/kg q 12–18 hr
  - 1,200–2,000 g, >7 days: 2.5 mg/kg q 8–12 hr
  - >2,000 g, 0–7 days: 2.5 mg/kg q 12 hr
  - >2,000 g, >7 days: 2.5 mg/kg q 8 hr
- Infants: 7.5–10 mg/kg/day/divided 8–12 hourly.

Brands: 10, 25, 50, 100, 200, 300 mg/vial; Netilmicin and Netromycin.

SISOMYCIN

Uses: Active against *Pseudomonas,* beta-hemolytic streptococci and other gram-negative bacilli.

Dosage:
- IV/IM: 1-2 mg/kg every 8 hourly.
- Eye drops: Instill 1-2 drops 4 hourly.

Brands: 10, 50 mg injection; Ensamycin, Sisoptin. 0.3% drop; Ensamycin, Sisocin.

STREPTOMYCIN

Uses: Used in combination therapy of active TB and in combination with other agents for treatment of streptococcal or enterococcal endocarditis.

Dosage: IM
- Neonates: 10–20 mg/kg/day
- Children: 20–40 mg/kg/day divided 12 hourly or single dose; not to exceed 1 g/day.

Brands: 0.75 g, 1 g/vial; Ambistryn-S.

Administration: Select large muscle for IM; concentration not to exceed 500 mg/mL; rotate injection sites.

TOBRAMYCIN

Uses: Active against gram-negative bacilli, especially *E. coli, Enterobacter, Klebsiella, Serratia, Proteus* and *Pseudomonas*; ophthalmic infections.

Dosage: IV/IM
- Neonates:
  - PNA <7 days: 1,200–2,000 g : 2.5 mg/kg q 12–18 hr; >2,000 g: 2.5 mg/kg q 12 hr
  - PNA >7 days: 1,200–2,000 g: 2.5 mg/kg q 8–12 hr; >2,000 g: 2.5 mg/kg q 8 hr
- Children: 5–7.5 mg/kg/day
  - 0.3% ophthalmic solution: 1–2 drops every 1–4 hour depending upon severity of infection
  - 0.3% ophthalmic ointment: Apply 0.5" ribbon 2–3 times/day.

Brands: 20, 60, 80 mg/vial; Tobacin, Tobasafe, Tocin. 0.3% eye ointment and drops; Optob, Teflin, Tycin.

Administration: Final concentration should not exceed 10 mg/mL.
- With concomitant indomethacin use, increase dosing intervals.

CARBAPENEM

These agents exhibit their bactericidal activity by binding to penicillin-binding proteins; resulting in inhibition of growth and also results in damage to the cell wall thus causing cell lysis and death. Active against gram-positive and gram-negative aerobic and anaerobic bacteria. Not effective against methicillin-resistant *Staphylococcus aureus*. Co-administration with probenecid causes delayed excretion.

ERTAPENEM

Uses: Active against community infections caused by extended spectrum β-lactamase (ESBL) producing bacteria including *E.coli* and *Klebsiella*.

Dosage: IV: 30 mg/kg divided every 12 hourly (maximum dose : 1 g). Not recommended in <3 months of age.

Brands: 1 g Injection; Alerta, Ertacrit, Zivator.
- Administer reconstituted solution within 6 hours.

IMIPENEM

Uses: Active against gram-positive cocci and gram-negative bacilli including *P. aeruginosa* and anaerobes.

Dosage:
- Neonates: IV, IM
  - PNA ≤7 days: <1,200 g: 20 mg/kg divided q 18–24 hr; >1,200 g: 40 mg/kg/day divided q 12 hr
  - PNA >7 days: 1,200–2,000 g: 40 mg/kg/day divided q 12 hr; >2,000 g: 60 mg/kg/day divided q 12 hr
- Children: 60–100 mg/kg/day divided q 6–8 hr

Brands: 500, 1,000 and 1,500 mg injection; Primaxin (equivalent to 250, 500 and 750 mg respectively).

Administration: IV—final concentration should not exceed 5 mg/mL:
- Seizures may occur when used in patients with CNS infection. Pseudomembranous colitis may occur.

MEROPENEM

Uses: Active against gram-positive and gram-negative aerobic and anaerobic pathogens including *S. aureus, S.pneumoniae, H. influenzae, N. meningitidis, E. coli, Klebsiella,* etc.

Dosage:
- Neonates: IV
  PNA 0–7 days: 20 mg/kg/dose q 12 hr
  PNA >7 days: 20 mg/kg/dose q 8–12 hr.
- Children: 60 mg/kg/day divided q 8 hr; meningitis: 120 mg/kg/day divided q 8 hr (maximum: 6 g/day).

Brands: 500 and 1,000 mg injection; Meronem and Ronem.

Administration: Concentrations should not exceed 50 mg/mL.

CEPHALOSPORINS

Acts by binding to penicillin-binding proteins and inhibiting bacterial cell wall synthesis, resulting in cell lysis and death. Active against both gram-negative and gram-positive but as we move to higher generation, activity against gram negative goes on decreasing. Probenecid may decrease their renal tubular secretion and increases serum concentration. Third generation are highly resistant to β-lactamase. None of the currently available cephalosporins have good activity against *Enterococcus, Mycoplasma, Camplylobacter, Listeria* and *Clostridium difficile*.

CEFADROXIL

Uses: Streptococcal pharyngitis, tonsillitis; soft tissue infection (SSTI) caused by streptococci or staphylococci, urinary tract infection (UTI) caused by *Klebsiella, E. coli* and *Proteus mirabilis*.

Dosage: 30 mg/kg/day divided q 12 hr PO (maximum: 2 g/day).

Brands: 500 mg capsule; 125, 250, 500 mg tablet; 125 mg/5 mL suspension; Bludrox, Cefadrox, Cefadur, Droxyl, etc.

CEFAZOLIN

Uses: Treatment of respiratory tract, SSTI, UTI, biliary tract, bone and joint infections; and septicemia due to susceptible gram-positive cocci (except *Enterococcus*), preoperative prophylaxis; bacterial endocarditis prophylaxis for dental and upper respiratory tract procedure.

Dosage: IV/IM
- Neonates:
  - PNA <7 days: 40 mg/kg/day divided q 12 hr
  - PNA >7 days: <2,000 g: 40 mg/kg/day divided q 12 hr; >2,000 g: 60 mg/kg/day divided q 8 hr.

- Infants and children: 50–100 mg/kg/day divided q 8 hr (maximum: 6 g/day).
- Bacterial endocarditis prophylaxis for dental and upper respiratory procedures in penicillin allergic patients: 25 mg/kg 30 minutes before procedure (maximum: 1 g).

Brands: 250, 500, 1,000 mg/vial; Cezolin, Orizolin, Reflin.

CEFACLOR

Uses: *S. aureus, S. pneumoniae, H. influenzae*; treatment of otitis media, sinusitis and SSTI, bone, and joint infections; UTI caused by *E. coli, Klebsiella* and *Proteus*.

Dosage: 20–40 mg/kg/day divided q 8–12 hr PO; (maximum: 2 g). Twice daily option is for otitis media and pharyngitis.

Brands: 250, 500 mg capsule; 125, 250 mg tablet; 125 mg/5 mL syrup; Distaclor, Keflor.

CEFDITOREN PIVOXIL

Uses: Active against Group A *Staphylococcus haemolyticus*, also active against many gram-negative and gram-positive bacteria except *Pseudomonas aeruginosa* and *S. typhi*.

Dosage: PO— 9 mg/kg/day divided every 8 hourly.

Brands: 50, 200 mg tablet; 100 mg/5 mL syrup; Cefditoren, Spectoren, Torcef-O, Zostum-O.

CEFUROXIME

Uses: Staphylococci, Group B streptococci, pneumococci, *H. influenzae (type A and B), E. coli, Enterobacter,* and *Klebsiella*; treatment of upper respiratory tract infection (URTI) and lower respiratory tract infections (LRTI), otitis media, acute bacterial sinusitis, UTI, SSTI, bone and joint infection, and sepsis.

Dosage
- IV/IM—neonates: 40–100 mg/kg/day divided q 12 hr. 200–240 mg/kg/day divided q 8 hr.

- PO: Infants and children; pharyngitis, tonsillitis: 20–30 mg/kg/day divided q 8 hr (maximum: 500 mg/day). Acute otitis media, acute bacterial sinusitis; impetigo: 30 mg/kg/day divided q 8 hr (maximum: 1 g/day). Adolescents: Uncomplicated UTI: 125–250 mg q 12 hr; uncomplicated gonorrhea: Single 1 g dose.

Brands: 125, 250, 500 mg tablet; 125 mg/5 mL suspension; 250, 750 mg/vial; Altacef, Cetil, Zocef, etc.

Administration: >30 mg/mL for IV and should be administered over 15–30 minutes. For intravenous push administer over 3–5 minutes at a maximum concentration of 100 mg/mL.

CEFOTAXIME

Uses: LRTI, SSTI, bone and joint, intra-abdominal and genitourinary tract infections; Meningitis due to susceptible organisms, such as *H. influenzae* and *N. meningitidis; Neisseria gonorrhoeae*, etc.

Dosage: IM/IV
- Neonates:
  - <1,200 g: 100 mg/kg/day divided q 12 hr
  - 1,200–2,000 g: 100–150 mg/kg/day divided q 8–12 hr.
- Infants and children 1 month to 12 years:
  - <50 kg: 100–200 mg/kg/day divided q 6–8 hr. 200 mg/kg/day divided q 6 hr
  - >50 kg: Moderate to severe infection: 1–2 g q 6–8 hr; life-threatening infection: 2 g/dose q 4 hr (maximum: dose: 12g/day).

Brands: 125, 250, 500, 1,000 mg/vial; C-Tax, Omnicef, Taxim, Udicef.

Administration: In a concentration ranging from 20–100 mg/mL over a period of 5–30 minutes. For IM 250 mg/mL.

CEFTRIAXONE

Uses: Treatment of sepsis, meningitis, LRTI, SSTI, bone and joint, intra-abdominal and UTI. Active against H.influenzae, Neisseria and enterobacteriaceae; gonococcal infection or chancroid; periorbital or buccal cellulitis, salmonellosis or shigellosis, pneumonia of unestablished etiology (<5 years of age), otitis media, etc.

Dosage: IM/IV
- Neonates:
  - <2,000 g : 50 mg/kg/day q 24 hr
  - >2,000 g : 50–75 mg/kg/day q 24 hr.
- Gonococcal infection: 25–50 mg/kg/day q 24 hr for 7 days
- Infants and children: 50–75 mg/kg/day devided q 12–24 hr
- Meningitis: 80–100 mg/kg/day divided q 12–24 hr loading dose of 75 mg/kg may be administered at the start of therapy (maximum: dose: 4g/day).
- Chancroid: IM, 50 mg/kg as a single dose (maximum: dose: 250 mg).
- Acute epididymidis: IM, 250 mg in a single dose
- Acute otitis media: 50 mg/kg in a single dose (maximum 1 g)

Brands: 125, 250, 500, 1,000 g/vial; C-Tri, Cefaxone, Monocef.

Combinations: Ceftriaxone + Sulbactam.

Administration: Use Cefotaxime in place of ceftriaxone in hyperbilirubinemic neonates. IV push, over 2–4 minutes at a maximum concentration of 40 mg/mL. For IM 250 mg/mL.

CEFOPERAZONE

Uses: RTI, SSTI, UTI and sepsis. Active against *E. coli, Klebsiella* and *Haemophilus* but variable activity against *Streptococcus* and *Staphylococcus* species.

Dosage: IV/IM
- Neonates: 100 mg/kg/day divided q 12 hr
- Children: 100–150 mg/kg/day divided q 12 hr (maximum 12 g/day).

Brands: 250, 500, 1,000 mg/vial; Magnamycin, Myticef.

Combinations: Cefoperazone + Sulbactam.

Administration: For IM >250 mg/mL and IV 5–50 mg/mL over 30 minutes.
- Concomitant use of anticoagulants may increase the risk of severe hemorrhage. Cefoperazone may decrease vitamin K synthesis by suppressing gastrointestinal (GI) flora and vitamin 'K' deficiency may occur.

CEFTAZIDIME

Uses: RTI, UTI, SSTI, intra-abdominal, osteomyelitis, sepsis, and meningitis caused by enterobacteriaceae and *Pseudomonas*; empirical therapy for febrile, agranulocytopenic patients.

Dosage: IM/IV
- Neonates:
  - 1,200–2,000 g: 100 mg/kg/day divided q 12 hr
  - >2000 g: 150 mg/kg/day divided q 8 hr.
- Infants and children: 100–150 mg/kg/day divided q 8 hr.
- Meningitis: 150 mg/kg/day divided q 8 hr (maximum: 6 g/day).

Brands: 250, 500, 1,000 mg/vial; C-zid, Tizime, Zidime.

Administration: For IM >300 mg/mL and for IV 40–180 mg/mL.

CEFDINIR

Uses: Respiratory tract, SSTI and otitis media (OM); susceptible organisms are *S. pneumoniae, H. influenzae, M. catarrhalis* and *S. aureus*, etc.

Dosage: PO—children >6 months to 12 years: 14 mg/kg/day divided q 12 hr for 5–10 days in OM, pharyngitis/tonsillitis, SSTI, acute maxillary sinusitis (maximum: 600 mg/day).

Brands: 125 mg tablet; 300 mg capsule; 125 mg/5 mL suspension; Aldinir, Rtist, Sefdin.

- Administer with food, administer at least 2 hourly before or after antacids or iron supplements (as they decrease absorption by 40% and 80% respectively).

CEFEPIME

Uses: LRTI, SSTI, UTI by various gram-positive and gram-negative organisms.

Dosage: IV/IM: 100–150 mg/kg/day divided q 8–12 hr.

Brands: 500 mg, 1 and 2 g/vial; Cepime, Kefage, Novapime.

Administration: 40–100 mg/mL for IV and 300 mg/mL for IM.

- Not compatible with metronidazole, vancomycin, aminoglycosides, and aminophylline.

CEFIXIME

Uses: UTI, OM, RTI; susceptible organisms are *Streptococcus, H. influenzae, M. catarrhalis, N. gonorrhoeae*, etc.

Dosage: PO— 8 mg/kg/day divided q 12 hr (maximum: 400 mg/day). Enteric fever: 20 mg/kg/day q 12 hr for 7 days. Shigellosis: 8 mg/kg/day q 12 hr for 5 days. UTI: 16 mg/kg/day q 12 hr on day 1, then 8 mg/kg/day for 13 days.

Brands: 100, 200 mg tablet; 50 mg/5 mL suspension; Cefi, Cefspan, *Extacef*, Fixx.

- Cefixime may increase warfarin (increase PT) and carbamazepine levels.

CEFPODOXIME

Uses: Pneumonia, uncomplicated gonorrhea, SSTI, acute otitis media (AOM), pharyngitis, tonsillitis, UTI; active against *S. aureus, Streptococcus, H. influenzae, N. gonorrhoeae, E. coli, Klebsiella* and *Proteus*.

Dosage: PO– 10 mg/kg/day divided q 12 hr (maximum: 400 mg/day), Uncomplicated gonorrhea: 200 mg single dose.

Brands: 50, 100, 200 mg tablet; 50 and 100 mg/5 mL suspension; Cepodem, Doxcef, Monocef-O:

- Serum levels and absorption is reduced by antacids and H2-receptor antagonists.

CEFPROZIL

Uses: RTI, SSTI, OM; active against *S. aureus, Streptococcus, H. influenzae, E. coli, Klebsiella* and *Proteus*.

Dosage: PO– 30 mg/kg/day divided q 8–12 hr (maximum: 1 g/day). Pharyngitis/tonsillitis: 15 mg/kg/day q 12 hr. SSTI: 20 mg/kg once daily.

Brands: 250, 500 mg tablet; Refzil-O, Zemetril. 125, 250 mg/5 mL suspension; Refzil-O.

CEFTIBUTEN

Uses: Active against gram-positive and gram-negative bacteria except *Pseudomonas aeruginosa, Enterococcus,* and *Enterobacter.*

Dosage: PO— 9 mg/kg/day once daily.

Brands: 400 mg capsule; 90 mg/mL suspension; Procadex.

CEFTIZOXIME

Uses: UTI, SSTI, RTI, sepsis; active against gram-positive and gram-negative infections.

Dosage: IV/IM: >6 months of age and children: 30–60 mg/kg/day q 6–8 hr. In severe infections, up to 100–150 mg/kg/day.

Brands: 250 mg, 1 g/vial; Cefizox, Eldcef.

Administration: 50 mg/mL for IV.

- Sodium content of 1 g ceftizoxime is 60 mg (2.6 mEq).

CEFPIROME

Uses: Gram-positive, active against *Pseudomonas*, staphylococci, *Enterococcus*; UTI, LRTI, SSTI, septicemia, etc.

Dosage: IV/IM: 30–60 mg/kg/day divided q 12 hr.

Brands: 250, 500 mg tablet; Refzil-O, Zemetril. 125 mg, 250 mg/5 mL suspension; Refzil-O.

CEPHALEXIN

Uses: Group A-β-haemolytic *Streptococcus, Staphylococcus, Klebsiella pneumonia, E. coli* and *Proteus*. Used to treat RT, SSTI, bone and joint, genitourinary and otitis media.

Dosage: PO: 25–100 mg/kg/day divided q 6–8 hr (maximum: 4 g/day).

Brands: 250 and 500 mg capsule; 125 and 250 mg tablet; 125 and 250 mg/5 mL suspension; 100 mg/mL drops; Ceff, Nufex, Phexin, Sporidex.

LINCOSAMIDES

Acts by inhibiting RNA-dependent protein synthesis by binding to 50S ribosomal subunits, inhibiting peptide bond formation of susceptible organisms. Rapid infusion of undiluted lincosamides has led to cardiac arrest; pseudomembranous colitis, Stevens-Johnson syndrome (SJS), skin rashes, eosinophilia. Potentiates action of neuromuscular blocking agents.

CLINDAMYCIN

Uses: Active against aerobic gram-positive staphylococci and streptococci; *Fusobacterium, Bacteroids and Actinomyces*. Also has activity against Plasmodium, *Pneumocystis,* and Toxoplasma species.
- Topically for acne vulgaris.
- Cerebral and ocular toxoplasmosis.
- Adjunctive therapy for falciparum malaria.

Dosage:
- PO: 10–30 mg/kg/day divided q 6 hr (maximum: 1.8 g/day)
- IV/IM: 25–40 mg/kg/day divided q 6–8 hr (maximum: 4.8 g/day).
- Falciparum malaria: 20 mg/kg/day for 5 days.

Brands: 150, 300 mg capsule; 50 mg/mL injection; Clinan, Dalacin C. 1% cream; Acnecin, Mimosee.

LINCOMYCIN

Uses: URTI and osteomyelitis. Topically for acne vulgaris.

Dosage: PO: 30–60 mg/kg/day divided q 8 hr. IV/IM:10–20 mg/kg/day divided q 8–12 hr.

Brands: 250, 500 mg capsule; 125 mg/5 mL syrup; 300 mg/mL injection; Lycin and Lynx. 2% gel; Link and Lynx.

MACROLIDES

These are bacteriostatic agents and acts by suppression of RNA-dependent protein synthesis by reversibly binding to 50S subunit of 20S bacterial ribosomes. The macrolides have activities against susceptible strains of *Streptococcus pneumonia, Staphylococcus aureus* and *Staphylococcus pyogenus*. They are generally inactive against MRSA. Clarithromycin has superior gram positive activity and azithromycin have superior gram-negative activity when compared with erythromycin.

AZITHROMYCIN

Uses: Mild to moderate URTI and LRTI, pneumonia, SSTI, AOM, urethritis and cervicitis due to susceptible strain of *C. trachomatis, N. gonorrhoeae, M. catarrhalis, H. influenzae, S. aureus, S. pneumoniae, Mycoplasma, Streptococcus and Legionella*; endocarditis prophylaxis, *Salmonella*.

Dosage: PO/IV—Children >6 months:
- Respiratory tract infection (RTI): 10 mg/kg on day 1 (maximum: 500 mg/day) followed by 5 mg/kg/day once daily for 5 days (maximum: 250 mg/day)
- Otitis media: 10 mg/kg once daily for 3 days (maximum: 500 mg/day) or 10 mg/kg on day 1, followed by 5 mg/kg once daily for 2–5 days
- >2 years:
  - Pharyngitis, tonsillitis: 12 mg/kg once daily for 5 days (maximum: 500 mg/day)
  - Chancroid: Single dose of 20 mg/kg (maximum: 1 g).
  - Uncomplicated chlamydial trachomatis: Single dose of 20 mg/kg (maximum: 1 g)
  - Endocarditis prophylaxis: 15 mg/kg/dose 1 hour before procedure
  - Typhoid: 20 mg/kg/day.

Brands: 100, 250, 500 mg tablet; 100, 200 mg/5 mL suspension; ATM, Azithral, Zithrocin. 500 mg injection; Azithral.

Administration: Administer IV at a final concentration of 1–2 mg/mL over 1–3 hours.

CLARITHROMYCIN

Uses: URTI, LRTI, AOM, SSTI due to susceptible strains of *S.aureus, S.pyogenes, S.pneumoniae, H.influenzae, M. catarrhalis, Mycoplasma pneumoniae, C. trachomatis and Legionella* species; treatment of *H. pylori* infection; prophylaxis of bacterial endocarditis in penicillin allergic patients.

Dosage: PO
- Infants and children:
  - AOM: 15 mg/kg/day divided q 12 hr for 10 days
  - Respiratory, SSTI: 15 mg/kg/day divided 12 hourly for 7–14 days
  - Prophylaxis for bacterial endocarditis: 15 mg/kg 1 hourly before procedure.
- Adolescents: *H. pylori* (combination therapy with omeprazole or with bismuth subsalicylate, tetracycline and H_2-receptor antagonist) 250 mg twice, up to 500 mg 3 times/day.

Brands: 125, 250, 500 mg tablet; 125 mg/5 mL syrup; Clarie, Crixan, Maclar.

Concomitant use with terfenadine, astemizole, cisapride may result in QT interval prolongation, tachycardia, hypotension. Safety not established below 6 months of age. Clarithromycin increases serum levels of theophylline, carbamazepine, digoxin, cisapride.

ERYTHROMYCIN

Uses: URTI, LRTI, pharyngitis, skin infections due to streptococci and staphylococci; mycoplasma, *Legionella*, diphtheria, pertussis, cholera, acne, chancroid; to improve feeding intolerance in preterm infants.

Dosage: PO
- Neonate: <7 days: 20 mg/kg/day divided q 12 hr. >7 days: 30–40 mg/kg/day divided q 6–8 hr. Chlamydial pneumonia: 50 mg/kg/day divided q 6 hr for 14 days.
- Infants and children: 30–50 mg/kg/day divided q 6–8 hr (maximum: 2 g/day):
  - Chlamydial trachomatis: 50 mg/kg/day divided q 6 hr for 10–14 days
  - Feeding intolerance: 5 mg/kg/dose q 6 hr
  - Cholera: 40 mg/kg/day along with other antimicrobials
  - Diphtheria: 40–50 mg/kg/day along with antitoxin therapy for 14 days
  - Pertussis: 40–50 mg/kg/day for 14 days
  - Rheumatic fever prophylaxis: 250 mg twice daily in penicillin allergic patients.

Brands: 125, 250 mg tablet; 125 mg/5 mL syrup; Althrocin, Erythrocin. 3% Erytop cream and lotion for topical application in acne.

- Erythromycin decreases clearance of carbamazepine, cisapride, theophylline, digoxin and may lead to their toxicity (do not use it concurrently). Avoid milk and acidic beverages 1 hour before or after a dose; administer after food to decrease GI discomfort. Associated with hypertophic pyloric stenosis in young infants.

ROXITHROMYCIN

Uses: Respiratory, ear, nose, and throat (ENT), SSTI, genital tract infection caused by *Staphylococcus, Streptococcus, Corynebacterium, Listeria, Legionella, Mycoplasma*.

Dosage: PO: 5–8 mg/kg/day in divided doses 12 hourly.

Brands: 50 mg and 150 mg tablet; 50 mg/5 mL syrup; Arbid, Roxid, Roxe.

PENICILLINS

Acts by binding to bacterial cell wall resulting in cell lysis. Penicillins are the drug of choice for infection caused by group-A and group-B *Sreptococcus, T. pallidium, L. monocytogenus* and *N. meningitidis*. Semisynthetic ones (cloxacillin, dicloxacillin) are active against Staphylococcal infection (non-MRSA). The aminopenecillins (ampicillin, amoxicillin) has good activity against gram-negative organisms including *E. coli* and *H. influenzae*. The carboxypenicillins (ticacillin) and ureidopenicillins (piperacillin) have good activity against most strains of *P. aeruginosa*.

AMOXICILLIN

Uses: Active against *Salmonella, Shigella, Neisseria, E. coli, P. mirabilis, H. influenzae*. Used to treat OM, sinusitis, RTI, enteric fever, etc.

Dosage: PO
- Neonates: 20–30 mg/kg/day divided q 12 hr
- Infants and children: 20–50 mg/kg/day divided q 8–12 hr.
- AOM: 80–90 mg/kg/day

- Endocarditis prophylaxis: 50 mg/kg 1 hour before procedure
- Enteric fever: 100 mg/kg/day for 14 days.

Brands: 125 and 250 mg tablet; 250 and 500 mg capsule; 125 mg/5 mL syrup; 100 mg/mL drops; Novamox, Mox, Lamoxy.

AMOXICILLIN + CLAVULANIC ACID

Uses: Same as amoxicillin in addition β-lactamase-producing *M. catarrhalis, H. influenzae, Niesseria* and *S. aureus, Klebsiella*, etc.

Dosage (Amoxycillin base):
- Neonates: 30 mg/kg/day divided q 12 hr PO
- Infants and children: 20–45 mg/kg/day divided q 8–12 hr PO. 50–100 mg/kg/day divided q 6–8 hr IV.

Brands: 228.5 mg (200 + 28.5 mg), 375 mg (250 + 125 mg) and 625 mg (500 + 125mg) tablet; 228.5 mg (200+28.5 mg) and 157.2 mg (125 + 32.2 mg) suspension; 150 mg (125 + 25 mg), 300 mg (250 + 50 mg), 600 mg (500 + 100 mg), 1,200 mg (1 g + 200 mg) injection; Augmentin, Clavam.

AMPICILLIN

Uses: Active against Streptococci, Pneumococci, Enterococci, some strains of *H. influenzae, Salmonella, Shigella, E. coli* and *Klebsiella*.

Dosage: IV/IM–
- Neonates (Use 2 times the recommended doses for meningitis):
  - PNA <7 days: <2,000 g: 50 mg/kg/day divided q 12; >2,000 g: 75 mg/kg/day divided q 8 hr
  - PNA >7 days: <2,000 g: 75 mg/kg/day divided q 8 hr; >2,000 g: 100 mg/kg/day divided q 6 hr.
- Infants and children: 100–200 mg/kg/day divided q 6 hr. (for meningitis use twice the usual doses) maximum: 12 g/day
- Endocarditis prophylaxis: 50 mg/kg 30 minutes before procedure (maximum: 2 g).

Brands: 125 and 250 mg tablet; 250 and 500 mg capsule; 125 mg/5 mL suspension; 100 mg/mL drops; 250 and 500 mg injection; Ampillin, Aristocillin, Brodicillin, Roscillin.

Administration: For IV 30–100 mg/mL and can be given over 15–30 minutes. Do not give simultaneously with aminoglycosides.
- Chloroquine reduces ampicillin absorption. Probenecid increases ampicillin levels.

AMPICILLIN + SULBACTAM

Uses: Addition of Sulbactam enhances activity against penicillinase-producing bacteria, i.e., *S. aureus, Streptococcus, H. influenzae, E. coli, Klebsiella, B. fragilis*.

Dosage: Based on ampicillin component; IV/IM:
- Infants >1 month: 100–150 mg/kg/day divided q 6 hr
- Children: 100–200 mg/kg/day divided q 6 hr.

Brands: Ampicillin 1 g + Sulbactum 0.5 g/vial; Ampitum, Betamp, Sulbacin.

CARBENICILLIN

Uses: Active against susceptible strains of *P. aeruginosa, E. coli*, indole-positive *Proteus* and *Enterobacter*.

Dosage: IV/IM:
- Neonates:
  - PNA ≤7 day: <2,000 g: 225 mg/kg/day divided q 8 hr. >2,000 g: 300 mg/kg/day divided q 6 hr
  - PNA >7 day: 300–400 mg/kg/day divided q 6 hr.
- Children: 400–600 mg/kg/day divided q 4–6 hr.

Brands: 1 g and 5 g/vial; Carbelin, Pyoper.

CLOXACILLIN

Uses: Active against penicillinase-resistant *S. aureus* and other gram-positive cocci except *Enterococcus* and coagulase negative staphylococci.

Dosage: IV/PO—children >1 month: 50–100 mg/kg/day divided q 6 hr (maximum: 4 g/day).

Brands: 125 mg/5 mL syrup; 250 and 500 mg capsule; 250 and 500 mg injection; Biodox, Clocilin, Klox.

Combinations: Cloxacillin + Ampicillin.
- Loss of potency when mixed with Aminoglycosides and Polymixin-B

PENICILLIN G AQUEOUS (CRYSTALLINE PENICILLIN)

Uses: Active against most gram-positivecocci except *S. aureus*, some gram-negative organisms, such as *N. gonorrhoeae, N. meningitidis* and some anaerobes and *Spirochetes*.

Dosage: IV/IM
- Neonates: For meningitis use twice the usual doses:
  - PNA <7 days: 1.2–2 kg: 50,000 units/kg/day divided 12 hourly. >2 kg: 75,000 units/kg/day divided 8 hourly
  - PNA >7day: 1.2–2 kg: 75,000 units/kg/day divided 8 hourly. >2 kg: 100,000 units/kg/day divided 6 hourly.
- Children: 100,000–250,000 units/kg/day divided 4–6 hourly (maximum: 400,000 units/kg/day). Rheumatic fever prophylaxis and pneumococcal infections— 200,000 units bd.

Brands: Penicillin G sodium 500,000 and 10,00,000 units/ vial; Benzyl penicillin. Penicillin G potassium 200,000, 400,00 and 800,000 units tablet; Pentids.

Administration: For IV 100,000–500,000 units/mL and should be given over 30–60 minutes. For neonates, it is 50,000 units/mL. Do not administer orally along with meals.
- Use with caution in pre-existing seizure disorder. Penicillin G potassium content is 1.7 mEq/million units. Penicillin G sodium content is 2 mEq/million units.

PENICILLIN G BENZATHINE

Uses: Useful for treatment of infections responsive to persistent, low concentration of penicillin, e.g., *Streptococcus pharyngitis*, rheumatic fever prophylaxis.

Dosage: IM
- Neonates: >1.2 kg—50,000 units/kg once.
- Children: 300,000–1.2 million units/kg q 3–4 weeks (maximum:1.2–2.4 million units/dose).

Secondary rheumatic fever prophylaxis:

<6 years: 6,00,000 units q 3 weeks

>6 years: 12 lac units q 3 weeks.

Brands: 6, 12 and 24 lac units/vial; Longacillin, Penidura.

Administration: Do not give at the same site repeatedly as it may cause fibrosis and atrophy.

Use penicillin G benzathine and penicillin G procaine combination to achieve early peak levels in acute infections.

PENICILLIN G PROCAINE

Uses: Active against *T. pallidum* and organisms susceptible to low but prolonged serum levels.

Dosage: IM
- Neonates: >1.2 kg; 50,000 units/kg/day once
  (Avoid in this age group as sterile abscess and procaine toxicity may occur)
- Children: 25,000–50,000 units/kg/day divided q 12–24 hr (maximum: 4.8 million units/day).

Brands: Injection; Procaine penicillin 4,00,000 units/vial.

PENICILLIN V POTASSIUM

Uses: Active against most gram-positive cocci; *S. pneumoniae*, *Streptococcus* and some gram-negative bacteria *N. gonorrhoeae*, *N. meningitidis*.

Dosage: PO
- Children:
  - <12 years: 25–50 mg/kg/day divided q 6–8 hr (maximum: 3 g/day), >12 years: 125–500 mg q 6–8 hr.
  - Primary prevention of rheumatic fever: 250 mg 2–3 times/day for 10 days
  - Prophylaxis of pneumococcal infections in children with sickle cell disease:
  - <3 years: 125 mg bd, >3 years: 250 mg bd.

Brands: 125 mg and 250 mg tablet; Kaypen.
- Use with caution in patients with history of seizures. Each 250 mg penicillin V contain 0.7 mEq of potassium. Each 250 mg = 400,000 units of penicillin.

PIPERACILLIN

Uses: Active against *P. aeruginosa, E. coli, Serratia, Enterobacter* and *Bacteroids*.

Dosage: IV/IM
- Neonates:
  - PNA <7 days: 150 mg/kg/day divided q 8–12 hr. >7 day: 200 mg/kg/day divided q 6–8 hr.
- Children: 200–300 mg/kg/day divided q 4–6 hr.

Brands: 1 g and 2 g/vial; Pipralin, Piprapen.

Administration: For IV, 200 mg/mL can be given over 3–5 minutes.
- Sodium content of 1 g = 1.85 mEq.

PIPERACILLIN +TAZOBACTAM

Uses: Tazobactam expands activity of piperacillin against β-lactamase producing strains of *S. aureus, H. influenzae, B. fragilis, E. coli* and *Acinetobacter*.

Dosage: Based on piperacillin component:
- Infants: ≤6 months: 150–300 mg/kg/day divided q 6–8 hr
- Infants and childrens >6 months: 300–400 mg/kg/day divided q 6–8 hr

Brands: Available in 8:1 combination; 2.25 g (2 g + 250 mg) and 4.5 g (4 g + 500 mg) injection; Piptaz, Tazact, Torbac.

Administration: Can be given over 30 minutes at a maximum concentration of 200 mg/mL.

TICARCILLIN

Uses: Extended spectrum molecule active against *E. coli, Enterobacter, P. aeruginosa,* and *Bacteroides*.

Dosage: IV
- Neonates:
  - <2 kg: 150 mg/kg/day divided q 12 hr
  - >2 kg: 225 mg/kg/day divided q 8–12 hr.
- Infants and children: 200–300 mg/kg/day divided 4–6 hourly.

Brands: 3 and 5 g/vial; Ticanic.

Administration: Can be given IV at a maximum 100 mg/mL concentration over 30 minutes.
- Use with caution in patients with CHF due to high sodium content (1 g contain 5.2–6.5 mEq).

TICARCILLIN WITH CLAVULONIC ACID

Dosage: IV—200-300 mg/kg/day divided q 8 hourly.

Brands: 3 g ticarcillin + 100 mg clavulonic acid in 3.1 g injection; Cital, Megcillin, Ticarnic.

QUINOLONES

These act by affecting the function of two enzymes produced by bacteria, namely topoisomerase type IV and DNA gyrase; so that they can no longer repair DNA or help in its repair resulting in cell death.

CIPROFLOXACIN

Uses: Active against *Shigella, Salmonella, Neisseria, P. aeruginosa, Enterobacter, H. influenzae, S. aureus, Streptococcus.* Topically for corneal ulcers and conjunctivitis.

Dosage: PO—IV: Children: 15–30 mg/kg/day divided 12 hourly (maximum: PO—1.5 g/day. IV; 800 mg/day).
- *Contacts of N.meningitidis:* 20 mg/kg single dose.
- *Corneal ulcers:* Apply throughout the day and night. Two drops every 30 minutes, then gradually decrease the dose.
- *Superficial infection of eye:* 1-2 drops 4 times daily for 3-4 days.

Brands: 250, 500, 750 mg tablet; 2 mg/mL infusion; Alcipro, Cebran, Cifran, Ciplox. 3 mg/mL eye drops; Adiflox, Alcipro, Ciplox.

Administration: For IV it can be given over 30 minutes at a maximum concentration of 2 mg/mL.
- Use with caution in patients with seizures and renal problems. Avoid use along with dairy products, mineral supplements and antacids.

GATIFLOXACIN

Uses: Active against gram-positive, gram-negative pathogens; some anaerobes and atypical mycobacteria.

Dosage: 10 mg/kg/day single dose orally.

Brands: 200, 400 mg tablet; Gaity, Gatiquin, Zigat.

LEVOFLOXACIN

Uses: UTI, pneumonia, otitis media, SSTI.

Dosage: PO— IV (maximum dose: 500 mg/day):
- 6 months–<5 years: 10 mg/kg/dose twice daily
- 5–12 years: 10 mg/kg/dose twice daily.

Brands: 250, 500 mg tablet; 500 mg/mL injection; Glevo, L-cin, Levobact:
- Give IV over 1½ hour, rapid infusion may cause hypotension. Use with caution is diabetes, seizures, children <18 years.

MOXIFLOXACIN

Uses: Community acquired pneumonia, acute bacterial sinusitis, chronic bronchitis, SSTI. Conjunctivitis caused by susceptible strains of the aerobic gram-positive bacteria and aerobic gram-negative bacteria.

Dosage: PO/IV: 7.5–10 mg/kg once daily.
 Ophthalmic solution—1 drop every 8 hourly in each eye.

Brands: 4 mg tablet; Moxicip, Moxif, Stamox. 4 mg/mL infusion; M-Cin, Moxicip, Stamox. 0.5% eye drop; Apdrops, Milflox, Mosi.

NADIFLOXACIN

Uses: Acne vulgaris, folliculitis, sycosis vulgaris and other bacterial infection.

Dosage: Apply twice daily, for acne apply after washing the face.

Brands: 0.1% skin cream; Nadibact, Nadigrace, Nadimox.

NALIDIXIC ACID

Uses: Lower UTI caused by *E. coli*, *Enterobacter*, *Klebsiella* and *Proteus*.

Dosage: PO
- Children: >3 months: 50–55 mg/kg/day divided q 6 hr
- Prophylaxis of UTI: 25–30 mg/kg/day divided q 8 hr

Brands: 250, 500 mg tablet; 300 mg/5 mL syrup; Dix and Gramoneg.
- Avoid in children with Glucose-6-phosphate dehydrogenase (G6PD) deficiency and with history of seizures.

NORFLOXACIN

Uses: Primarily used for urinary and genital tract infections and bacterial diarrheas. Topically for eye and ear infections.

Dosage: PO: 6–12 mg/kg/day divided q 12 hr.

Brands: 100, 200, 400 mg tablet; Norbactin, Norbid, Utibid. 100 mg/5 mL suspension; Tamflox, Wyflox.
- Antacids interfere with absorption.

OFLOXACIN

Uses: Active against gram-positive, anaerobes and chlamydia. Useful for corneal ulcers, conjunctivitis, otitis externa, and chronic suppurative otitis media (CSOM).

Dosage:
- PO: 15 mg/kg/day divided q 12 hr
- IV: 5–10 mg/kg/day divided q 12 hr.

Brands: 200 and 400 mg tablet; 50 mg/5 mL suspension; 2 mg/mL infusion; Bioff, Oflox, Zanocin, Zenflox, etc., 0.3% eye drops; Atoflox, Entof, fuvid.

TETRACYCLINES

Tetracyclines are primarily bacteriostatic. These acts by inhibiting bacterial protein synthesis by binding to 30S ribosomes in susceptible organisms. Tetracyclines have a broad spectrum of activity that includes most *Rickettsia, Chlamydia, Mycoplasma* species, *Spirochetes* and some gram-negative and gram-positive bacteria. Must be prescribed judiciously to children <8 years of age because they can cause teeth staining, hypoplasia of dental enamel, and abnormal bone growth.

DEMECLOCYCLINE

Uses: Active against most gram-positive cocci except Enterococcus, many gram-negative bacilli, anaerobes, Mycoplasma, Chlamydia, and *Borrelia*.

Dosage: PO: 8–12 mg/kg/day divided q 6–12 hourly.

Brands: 150, 300 mg capsule; Ledermycin.

- Aluminium, calcium, magnesium, zinc, and iron containing food and drugs; milk and dairy products decreases absorption if given concurrently.

DOXYCYCLINE

Uses: Active against gram-positive cocci except *Enterococcus*, many gram-negative bacilli, anaerobes, *Mycoplasma* and *Chlamydia*.

Dosage: PO: 2–5 mg/kg/day divided q 12–24 hr (maximum: 200 mg/day). Cholera: 5 mg/kg single dose.

Brands: 100 and 200 mg tablet; Doxy-1, Vibazine.

- Contraindicated in children <8 years due to associated retardation in skeletal development, permanent discoloration of teeth, and enamel hypoplasia. Administration along with iron, calcium and milk decreases its absorption.

MINOCYCLINE

Uses: Active against *S. aureus, E. coli, Acinetobacter, K. pneumoniae, Serratia marcescens*.

Dosage: 4 mg/kg/day divided q 12 hr. Initially, followed by 2 mg/kg every 12 hr.

Brands: 50, 100 mg tablet; CNN and Minolin.

OXYTETRACYCLINE

Uses: External bacterial infection of eyes caused by susceptible organisms, trachoma.

Dosage: 1cm ribbon of ointment to be applied 2-3 times/day.

Brands: 10 mg/g ointment; Terramycin.

TETRACYCLINE

Uses: Treatment of Rocky Mountain spotted fever, acne vulgaris, lyme disease and mycoplasma disease.

Dosage: PO: 25–50 mg/kg/day divided q 6 hr (maximum: 3 g/day).

Brands: 250, 500 mg capsule; Hostacycline, Subamycin, Tetracycline.
- Administer 1 hourly before or 2 hourly after meals.

TIGECYCLINE

Uses: Active against Enterobacteriaceae, including extended spectrum β-lactamase producers, streptococci, staphylococci and anaerobes.

Dosage: IV—1.5 mg/kg as a loading dose (maximum 100 mg) followed by maintenance dose of 1 mg/kg/day (maximum 50 mg) divided 12 hourly infusion.

Brands: 50 mg/vial; Egytig, Tiganex, Tigimox.

MISCELLANEOUS ANTIMICROBIALS

AZTREONAM

Uses: UTI, LRTI, septicemia, SSTI, etc. Active against gram-negative aerobic bacteria, enterobacteriaceae, *Pseudomonas, H. influenzae*, etc.

Dosage: IV/IM

Neonates:
- PNA <7 days: <2,000 g: 60 mg/kg/day divided q 12 hr, >2000 g: 90 mg/kg/day divided q 8 hr.
- PNA >7 days: <2,000 g: 90 mg/kg/day divided q 8 hr, > 2,000 g: 120 mg/kg/day divided q 6–8 hr.
- Children: 90–120 mg/kg/day divided q 6–8 hr.

Brands: 0.5 g, 1 g and 2 g/vial; Azenam, Aztreo.

Administration: For IV 20–60 mg/mL; can be given over 10–60 minutes.
- Probenecid and furosemide increases serum levels.

CHLORAMPHENICOL

Uses: Active against *Bacteroides, H. influenzae, N. meningitidis, S. pneumoniae, Salmonella, Mycoplasma,* etc. Topically for conjunctivitis and otitis externa.

Dosage:
- Infants and children: 50–75 mg/kg/day divided q 6 hr IV or PO
- Meningitis: IV; infants and children: 75–100 mg/kg/day divided 6 hourly.
- Ocular: 1-2 drops 2-4 times /day.

Brands: 250, 500 mg capsule; 125 mg/5 mL suspension; 1 g/ vial; Enteromycetin, Paraxin. 1% eye drops; Andrecin, Chlormet, Paraxin.

Three major toxicities are aplastic anemia, bone marrow suppression and gray baby syndrome. Rifampicin, phenytoin, and phenobarbitone may increase serum levels. Use with caution in G6PD deficiency. May decrease absorption of vitamin B_{12}.

COLISTIMETHATE SODIUM

Uses: Active against gram-negative aerobic bacilli including *P. aeruginosa, E. coli, K. pneumoniae*.

Dosage: IV: 1,50,000 units/kg as loading dose then 12 hour later as 1,50,000 units/kg/day divided q 8 hourly.

Brands: 1,2 million units/vial; Xylistin, Acostin.
- Cause nephro- and neurotoxicity. Increased nephrotoxicity when used with diuretics.

COLISTIN SULFATE

Uses: For gram-negative bacillary diarrhea and pseudomonal enteritis.

Dosage: 5–15 mg/kg/day divided q 6–8 hr PO.

Brands: 12.5 mg/5 mL, 25 mg/5 mL suspension; Colistop, Gd safe, Walamycin.

DAPTOMYCIN

Uses: Active against methicillin-resistant *S. aureus* (MRSA), methicillin-susceptible *S. aureus* (MSSA), *S. aureus* and *Staphylococcus* species. Useful for skin and soft tissue infection, endocarditis, bacteremia.

Dosage: IV—skin and soft tissue infection: 4 mg/kg once daily for 7–14 days.
- Endocarditis and bacteremia: 6–8 mg/kg for 2–4 weeks.

Brands: 350 mg injection; Daptocure.
- Most significant side effects is elevation of creatine phosphokinase (CPK) and should be monitored weekly and drug should be stopped if CPK > 10 times normal.

FOSFOMYCIN

Uses: Active against gram-positive organisms (*E. faecalis, S. aureus, S. pneumoniae, S. epidermis*) and gram-negative pathogens (*Salmonella, Shigella, E. coli, Klebsiella, Enterobacter species*). Also active against some aerobes.

Dosage: PO/IV—Preterm: 50 mg/kg twice daily.
- Neonate: 60-70 mg/kg thrice daily.
- Children: 100 mg/kg thrice daily.

Brands: 3 g sachet; Fosirol, Monurol, Fosfocin. 4 g injection; Crifos, Fosfocin, Fosfotas.
- Sachet should be diluted in one cup of water. Severe side effects associated with IV use are—hypokalemia, hypernatremia, heart failure, hypertension (HT).

FURAZOLIDONE

Uses: For enteritis and protozoal diarrhea; active against *Salmonella, Shigella*, giardia, etc.

Dosage: Infants >1 month and children—PO—5–9 mg/kg/ day; divided q 6 hr (maximum: 400 mg).

Brands: 25 mg/5 mL syrup; 100 mg tablet; Furoxone.
- Avoid in G6PD deficiency. Use in infants <1 month may cause hemolytic anemia. Urine color is changed to orange during its use.

FUSIDIC ACID

Uses: Active against Staphylococci, Streptococci, *Corynebacterium* and other organisms.

Dosage: Apply twice or thrice daily for 5-7 days.

Brands: 2% ointment; Fucidin, Fusiderm, Fusiwal.

LINEZOLID

Uses: Treatment of pneumonia, SSTI, bacteremia caused by vancomycin-resistant *Enterococcus, Streptococcus pneumoniae*, *Staphylococcus aureus*, etc.

Dosage: Infants and children—IV or PO—10 mg/kg/dose q 8–12 hr.

Brands: 600 mg tablet; 2 mg/mL infusion; Linox, Lizolid, Lizomed.

Administration: For IV—infuse over 30–120 minutes.
- May cause pseudomembranous colitis and myelosuppression.

MUPIROCIN

Uses: Active against *Staphylococcs* and *Streptococcus*. Impetigo, folliculitis, furunculosis, infected dermatosis.

Dosage: Apply to affected area thrice daily. Nasal application: Apply to inner surface of each nostril 2–3 times/day for 5–7 days.

Brands: 2% ointment and cream; Bactroban, B-bact, Mupi.

NITROFURANTOIN

Uses: Prevention and treatment of UTI caused by *E. coli, Klebsiella, Enterobacter, S. aureus*, etc.

Dosage: Infants >1 month and children: 5–7 mg/kg/day divided q 6 hr (maximum: 400 mg/day). UTI prophylaxis: 1–2.5 mg/kg/day single dose (maximum: 100 mg/day).

Brands: 50 mg, 100 mg tablet; 25 mg/5 mL suspension; Furadantin.
- Should not be used to treat UTI in febrile infants and young children in whom renal involvement is likely. Use with caution in anemia, G6PD and vitamin B deficiency, DM, etc.

POLYMYXIN B SULFATE

Uses: Treatment of otitis externa. Rarely used parenteral for enteral and systemic infections.

Dosage:
- IV/IM: 15,000–25,000 units/kg/day divided q 12 hr (maximum: 2,000,000 units/day).
- Topical: 0.1%–0.3% solution.

Brands: 500,000 IV/vial; Aerosporin.

Administration: Infuse slowly at a concentration of 1,000– 1,600 units/mL.
- 1 mg of polymyxin B = 10,000 units. IM route is not recommended due to severe pain.
- Synergistic with cephalosporins. Increase nephrotoxicity with aminoglycosides.

RIFAXIMIN

Uses: Traveler's diarrhea, hepatic encephalopathy and *Clostridium difficile* infection.

Dosage: PO—children >12 years: 200 mg thrice daily for 3–7 days.

Brands: 200,400,550 mg tablet; Rifagut, Torfix, Rixmin.
- Side effects are black tarry stool, dizziness, muscle spasm and trouble sleeping.

SILVER SUFADIAZINE

Uses: Various degree of burns and chronic ulcer.

Dosage: Apply thrice or four times daily. Frequency of reapplication is based on washing off due to patient activity or volume of exudates.

Brands: 1% cream; Siver sufadiazine, Silvindon.
- Discard 50 g tube 7 days after opening and 200 and 500 g pots 24 hour after opening.

TEICOPLANIN

Uses: Active againstgram-positive organisms only (staphylococci, streptococci, and enterococci).

Dosage: IM/IV—10 mg/kg 12 hourly. For 3 doses followed by 6–10 mg/kg/day.

Brands: 200 and 400 mg/vial; Targocid and Ticocin.
- Chances of auditory and vestibular changes with concomitant use with other ototoxic agents.

TRIMETHOPRIM + SULFAMETHOXAZOLE

Uses: Prophylaxis and treatment of *P. carinii* pneumonia; UTI caused by *E. coli, Klebsiella, P. mirabilis, Enterobacter*; susceptible shigellosis and typhoid.

Dosage: Children >2 months; PO:
- Mild to moderate infections: 6–12 mg of TMP/kg/day divided q 12 hr.
- Severe infection: 15–20 mg of trimethoprim (TMP)/kg/day divided q 6–8 hr.
- Prophylaxis of pneumocystis: 5 mg/kg of TMP single dose on alternate day
- UTI prophylaxis: 2 mg of TMP/kg/dose daily or 5 mg TMP/kg/dose twice weekly.

Brands: TMP + SMZ: 160 + 800 mg, 80 + 400 mg and 20 + 100 mg tablet; 40 + 200 mg/5 mL suspension; Bactrim, Septran. 160 mg + 800 mg table; Sepmax.
- Contraindication in folate deficiency megaloblastic anemia. May cause Stevens-Johnson syndrome, agranulocytosis, hepatic necrosis.
- Prolongs half life of phenytoin. Increase toxicity with concomitant use of other antifolate drugs.

VANCOMYCIN

Uses: Active against gram-positive pathogens including *Staphylococcus* (including MRSA and coagulase negative staphylococci), *S. pneumoniae, Enterococcus* and *Clostridium difficile* associated colitis.

Dosage: IV
- Neonates:
  - PNA <7 days: 1,200–2,000 g: 15 mg/kg/day divided q 12–18 hr. >2,000 g: 30 mg/kg/day divided q 12 hr
  - PNA >7 days: 1,200–2,000 g: 15 mg/kg/day divided q 8–12 hr. >2,000 g: 45 mg/kg/day divided q 8 hr.

- Infants >1 month and children: 40–60 mg/kg/day divided q 6 hr (maximum: 1 g/dose).
- Clostridium associated colitis: PO—40–50 mg/kg/day divided q 6–8 hr.

Brands: 500 mg and 1 g vial; Vancocin CP and Vancogen. 125 mg capsule; Vancocin CP.

Administration: IV: Concentration should not exceed 5 mg/mL.
- Rapid infusion is associated with 'red man syndrome' administration of antihistamines just before infusion may prevent or minimize this reaction.
- Additive effects with other drugs causing nephro- and ototoxicity.

Anticoagulants

chapter 5

These drugs are used for the prevention and treatment of thromboembolic disorders. They prevent clot formation and extension but do not dissolve clots. Therapy is usually initiated with heparin because of rapid onset of action, while maintenance therapy consists of warfarin. Warfarin takes several weeks to produce therapeutic anticoagulation. These should be avoided in underlying coagulation disorders, ulcer disease, malignancy, recent surgery or active bleeding.

ENOXAPARIN

Uses: Treatment and prophylaxis of venous thromboembolism.

Dosage: SC—Prophylaxis: <2 months:1.5 mg/kg/day; >2 months:1 mg/kg/day in 2 divided doses (maximum: 40 mg/day).

- Treatment: <2 months: 3 mg/kg/day; >2 months: 2 mg/kg/day in 2 divided doses.

Brands: 20 mg injection; Clexane, LMWX. 40, 60 mg injection; CDPARIN, Enclex, LMWX.

May cause hemorrhage, thrombocytopenia, gastrointestinal (GI) symptoms. Do not rub after SC injection as bruising may occur. Therapy should be discontinued if platelet count falls below 1 lakh/mm^3. Accidental overdosage may be treated with protamine sulfate.

HEPARIN

Uses: Treatment and prophylaxis of thromboembolic disorders.

Dosage: IV

- Loading dose of 50 units/kg given over 10 minutes followed by continuous infusion of 15–35 units/kg/h as maintenance dose

- For arterial lines and total parenteral nutrition (TPN): 0.5–1 units/mL is added
- For line flushing: 10–100 units/mL (volume used is 2–5 mL/flush).
- For umbilical artery catheter: 0.25–1 unit/mL (maximum : 200 unit/day).

Brands: 1,000 and 5,000 units/mL injection; Beparine, Heparin, Vparin.
- To reverse the effect of heparin use protamine. Contraindicated in severe thrombocytopenia, bacterial endocarditis, intracranial hemorrhage, shock. Maintain activated partial thromboplastin time (APTT) to 1.5–2.5 times of control.

WARFARIN

Uses: Treatment and prophylaxis of venous thromboembolic and pulmonary embolism; arterial thromboembolism in patient with prosthetic heart valves or atrial fibrillation.

Dosage: PO—Loading dose of 0.2 mg/kg once then followed by 0.1 mg/kg/day. Dose is titrated according to prothrombin time value.

Brands: 1, 2 and 5 mg tablet; Uniwarfin, Warf.
- Overdose can be treated with vitamin K. May cause hemoptysis, hemorrhage, skin necrosis, GI symptoms.

Antidepressants

chapter 6

These drugs are used in the treatment of various forms of endogenous depression, often in conjunction with psychotherapy. These help by overall re-regulation of the abnormal receptor neurotransmitter relationship. Administer drugs that are sedative at bedtime to avoid excessive drowsiness during working hours, and administer drugs that cause insomnia in the morning.

AMITRIPTYLINE

Uses: Depression, migraine prophylaxis, analgesic for neuropathic pain, nocturnal enuresis.

Dosage: PO:
- Depression: 1–1.5 mg/kg/day divided q 8 hr
- Analgesic and migraine prophylaxis: 0.5 mg/kg at bedtime can be increased gradually over 2–3 week to 2 mg/kg at bedtime.
- Nocturnal enuresis: <2 years:10–25 mg and >2 years: 25–50 mg at bedtime for 8–10 weeks.

Brands: 10 mg, 25 mg, 50 mg tablet; Nildep, Tryptomer.
- May cause postural hypotension, drowsiness, confusion, constipation, weight gain, tremor, urine discoloration, blurred vision, dry mouth, urinary retention. Do not stop abruptly in patient on chronic therapy.

ARIPIPRAZOLE

Uses: Schizophrenia, autism spectrum disorder (ASD).

Dosage: PO–Schizophrenia: Children 15–18 years: 2 mg once daily, can be increased every 2 days to maximum of 30 mg/day.
- ASD: >6 years—2 mg/day can be increased gradually upto 5 mg/day.

Brands: 10, 25, 50 mg tablet; Arip, Amitone, Amypres.

BUPROPION

Use: Depression, attention deficit hyperactivity disorder (ADHD).

Dosage: PO: 75–100 mg/day in three divided doses.

Brands: 150 mg tablet; Bupep, Zyban.

DOXEPIN

Use: Depression, relief from neuropathic pain.

Dosage: 1–3 mg/kg/day in 1–2 divided doses.

Brands: 25 mg tablet; Dox, Saliter. 10, 25 and 75 mg capsule; Dox, Spectra.
- May cause excessive sedation, postural hypotension, anticholinergic effect.

FLUOXETINE

Use: Depression and obsessive-compulsive disorder.

Dosage: PO—children >5 years: 5–10 mg starting dose and can be gradually increased to maximum dose of 20 mg/kg/day once daily.

Brands: 10 and 20 mg tablet; Flunat, Flunil, Nuzac, Prodep.
- May cause headache, nervousness, anxiety, insomnia, diarrhea, anorexia, constipation. Evening dose can be given before 4 PM to avoid insomnia.

IMIPRAMINE

Uses: Depression, enuresis.

Dosage: PO
- Depression: 1.5 mg/kg/day, if required may be increased to 1 mg/kg every 3–4 days to a maximum of 5 mg/kg/day in divided doses.
- Enuresis: For children >6 years start at 10–25 mg at bedtime, if adequate response is not seen after 1 week then can be increased gradually to 50 mg; for 6–12 years of age and 75 mg for >12 years of age. Continue the dose at which the desired effect is achieved for 2–3 months, then taper slowly. When dry for 3 weeks give drug on alternate days for 2 weeks.

Brands: 25 mg tablet; 75 mg capsule; Antidep, Depsonil, Impramine.
- Side effect same as Amitriptyline.

LITHIUM

Use: Acute manic episodes, depression, bipolar disorders.

Dosage: PO—15–60 mg/kg/day in 3–4 divided doses (maximum: 900 mg/day). Start at lower doses and adjust weekly.

Brands: 250, 300, 400 mg tablet; Lithium, Lithosun. 150 mg tablet; Intalith.
- May cause polydipsia, weight gain, impaired taste, tremor, leukocytosis, vision problem, fatigue, hypotension, seizures.

NORTRIPTYLINE

Uses: Antidepressant, nocturnal enuresis.

Dosage: PO
- Depression: 1–3 mg/kg/day divided q 6 hr
- Nocturnal enuresis: 10–20 mg/day, titrate upward to a maximum of 40 mg/day. Give dose 30 minutes before bedtime

Brands: 25 mg tablet; Daventyl, Nordep, Sensival.
- May cause postural hypotension, tachycardia, weight gain, xerostomia, urinary retention, tremor, blurred vision.

SERTRALINE

Uses: Depression, obsessive-compulsive disorder, panic disorder, attention deficit disorder, post-traumatic stress disorder.

Dosage: PO
- 6–12 years: Initial 25 mg/day, can be increased by 25 mg weekly up to a desired response (maximum: 200 mg/day)
- >12 years: Initial 50 mg/day, increase 25–50 mg weekly up to a desired response (maximum: 200 mg/day).

Brands: 25, 50 and 100 mg tablet; Serlift, Serne, Serta, Setral.
- May cause dry mouth, gastrointestinal (GI) disturbances, tremor, insomnia, fatigue, urinary incontinence.

Antidotes/Poisoning

chapter 7

A poison has been defined as a substance which when introduced into or absorbed by a living organisms, causes injury or death. Thus a variety of substances may act as a poison including the medicines. Children are the most vulnerable section of our society and one of the principle victim of poisoning. Childhood poisoning involve accidental ingestion in toddlers and preschool children falling prey to their own curiosity; to intentional overdoses in the adolescents. Poisoning is more common in male children; and there is a higher incidence in lower economic strata of society. The present day household, offer toxic substances at every corner of house including caustics, insecticides and medicines which are easily approachable to children. There are only very few specific antidotes available; other only modify the symptoms.

ACETYLCYSTEINE

Uses: Acetaminophen (paracetamol) toxicity.

Dosage: PO– initial dose of 140 mg/kg followed by 70 mg/ kg q 4 hr for 68 hours (17 doses). IV– initial dose of 150 mg/kg over ½–1 hr followed by 50 mg/kg over 4 hours, then 100 mg/kg over 16 hours.

Brands: 600 mg tablet; 200 mg/mL solution (20%) for injection; Mucomix.

- Acute flushing and erythema may occur within ½–1 hour after IV infusion. Use with caution in patient with asthma or prior history of bronchospasm.

ATROPINE

- *Refer* Chapter 3 'Antiarrhythmics'.

BENZTROPINE

Uses: Treatment of drug-induced extrapyramidal effects and acute dystonic reaction.

Dosage: 0.02–0.05 mg/kg/dose bd; IV or PO in children >3 years of age (maximum: 4 mg).

Brands: 0.5 and 1 mg tablet; 1 mg/mL injection; Cogentin.

Side effect: Sedation, blurred vision, dry mouth, tachycardia.

CYANIDE KIT (AMYL NITRITE, SODIUM NITRITE, SODIUM THIOSULFATE)

Uses: Cyanide and hydrogen sulfide (nitrite only) poisoning.

Dosage:
- Amylnitrite: 0.3 mL inhalation for 15–30 seconds of each minute followed by rest
- Sodium nitrite: 0.33 mL/kg of 3% solution slowly IV (maximum: 10 mL)
- Sodium thiosulfate: 1.65 mL/kg of 25% solution IV at a rate of 2.5–5 mL/minute (maximum: 50 mL).

Side effect: Methemoglobinemia (avoid levels > 30%).

CHARCOAL

Refer 'Miscellaneous Drugs'.

CHLORPROMAZINE

Uses: Amphetamine toxicity.

Dosage: IM, IV– 1 mg/kg (maximum dose 50 mg).

Brands: 25 mg/mL injection; Megatil.

DEFERIPRONE

Refer Chapter 27 'Chelating Agents'.

DESFERRIOXAMINE

Refer Chapter 27 'Chelating Agents'.

DIGOXIN IMMUNE FAB

Uses: Digitalis glycoside toxicity.

Dosage: IV—Depends upon body load of digoxin, it can be determined as milligram of digoxin ingested × 0.8. One vial binds 0.6 mg of digitalis glycoside.

Brands: 38 mg/vial; Digibind.

DIMERCAPROL (BAL)

Refer Chapter 27 'Chelating Agents'.

DIMERCAPTOSUCCINIC ACID (SUCCIMER, DMSA)

Uses: Lead poisoning.

Dosage: PO—10 mg/kg/dose q 8 hr for 5 days, then 10 mg/kg 12 hours.

Brands: 100 mg capsule; Chemet.

DIPHENHYDRAMINE

Uses: Phenothiazine-induced dystonic reactions.

Dosage: PO—5 mg/kg/day divided q 8 hr (maximum: 300 mg/day).

Brands: 12.5 mg/5 mL syrup; Benadryl.

Side effects: Sedation, paradoxical agitation, ataxia.

D-PENICILLAMINE

Refer Chapter 27 'Chelating Agents'.

EDETATE CALCIUM DISODIUM (CALCIUM EDTA)

Uses: Lead, manganese, nickel and zinc toxicity.

Dosage: IM, IV—50–75 mg/kg/day or 1–1.5 g/m^2/day divided q 6 hr as 0.2%–0.4% solution for 5 days.

Brands: Available as 200 mg/mL injection.

- IM route is preferred over IV. Avoid rapid IV infusion as it may lead to fatal elevation of ICP. May cause hypertension (HT), allergic reaction, nephrotoxicity.

ETHANOL

Uses: Ethylene glycol and methyl alcohol ingestion.

Dosage:
- Ethylene glycol ingestion: 10 mL/kg of 10% solution IV or 1 mL/kg of 95% solution PO; maintenance dose is 1.5 mL/kg/h of 10% solution IV or 3 mL/kg/h of 10% solution during hemodialysis.
- Methanol ingestion: 10 mL/kg of 10% solution IV as loading dose followed by 1.5 mL/kg/h infusion
- Target of treatment is to achieve methanol/ethylene glycol blood level of 100–130 mg/dL.

FLUMAZENIL

Uses: Benzodiazepine toxicity.

Dosage: IV– given in incremental doses of 0.1, 0.2, 0.3 mg at 1 minute interval until desired effect is achieved (maximum: 1 mg).

Brands: 0.1 mg/mL in 5 and 10 mL vials; Anexate.
- Do not use in unknown or antidepressant ingestion.

GLUCAGON

Refer 'Miscellaneous Drugs'.

HYPERBARIC OXYGEN

Uses: Carbon monoxide poisoning.

Dosage: Half-life of carboxyhemoglobin is 5 hours in room air, but in 100% oxygen half-life is 1.5 hours. Give until carboxyhemoglobin level comes to <10%.

METHYLENE BLUE

Uses: Methemoglobinemia (drug induced).

Dosage: IV—0.1–0.2 mL/kg of 1% solution by slow infusion, may be repeated after 30–60 minutes if methemoglobin level remains greater than 30%.

Brand: Available as 10 mg/mL injection; Bluejet.

NALOXONE

Uses: Morphine and other opioid poisoning.

Dosage: IV– 0.1 mg/kg/dose may be repeated q 2–3 minutes if required till the reversal of toxic effect (maximum: 2 mg/dose and total maximum: 10 mg).

Brands: 0.4 mg/mL injection; Nalox, Narcotan.

OCTREOTIDE

Uses: Sulfonylurea poisoning.

Dosage: IV—1 µg/kg/dose q 12 hr.

Brands: 50 and 100 µg/mL injection; Actide, Octate.

- During octreotide therapy, also required simultaneously high dose glucose.

PHYSOSTIGMINE

Uses: Anticholinergic stress (*Dhatura* poisoning), baclofen and atropine toxicity.

Dosage: IM, IV– 0.02 mg/kg, may be repeated q 5–10 minutes to maximum 2 mg or till the desired effect occur.

- May cause bradycardia, asystole, seizure.

PILOCARPINE

Use: Atropine toxicity.

Dosage: 2–4 mg, PO.

Brand: 10 mg tablet; Pilomax.

PRALIDOXIME (PAM)

Use: Organophosphorus (insecticide) poisoning.

Dosage: IM/IV– 25–50 mg/kg as 5% solution over 15–20 minutes. The dose may be repeated after 1–2 hr and then at 10–12 hr interval if cholinergic crisis recur.

Brands: 1 mg injection; Clopam, Lyphe.

Side effects: Tachycardia, bronchospasm, seizure.

PROTAMINE
Refer Chapter 'Drug Used for Controlling Bleeding'.

PRAZOCIN
Uses: Scorpion bite.

Dosage: PO– 0.25 mg every 4–6 hourly for 24 hours.

Brands: 1,2 tablet; Prazopress. 2.5, 5 *mg* tab; Prazopress XL, Minipress XL.

PYRIDOXINE
Refer Chapter 47 'Vitamins'.

VITAMIN K (PHYTOMENADIONE)
Uses: Warfarin poisoning.

Dosage: 5–10 mg IM or IV.

Brand: 10 mg/mL injection; Kenadion.

ADDITIONAL ANTIDOTES

Calcium gluconate: Used in calcium channel blocker overdose and in hydrofluoric acid poisoning

D-25 and 50%: Used in insulin overdoses

Edrophonium, neostigmine: Used in neuromuscular-blocking agent poisoning

Sodium bicarbonate: Phenothiazine and tricyclic antidepressant poisoning

Calcium folinate: Methotrexate, pyrimethamine, trimethoprim toxicity.

Antiemetics

These agents are used to manage nausea and vomiting of various etiology including infection, surgery, anesthesia, antineoplastic, and radiation therapy. The underlying cause of the symptoms must be elicited before emesis is corrected because antiemetics may mask signs of underlying pathology or overdosage of other drugs.

DIMENHYDRINATE

Uses: Prevention and treatment of nausea, vomiting, and vertigo associated with motion sickness.

Dosage: PO, IV, IM– not indicated below 2 years.
- 2–5 years: 12.5–25 mg q 6–8 hr (maximum: 75 mg/day)
- 6–12 years: 25–50 mg q 6–8 hr (maximum: 150 mg/day).

Brands: 50 mg tablet; Draminate, Gravol. 15.6 mg/5 mL syrup; 50 mg/mL injection; Draminate.
- May cause excitation in young children; use with precautions in patients with seizure disorder. May lead to masking of signs and symptoms of ototoxicity in patients on aminoglycosides, furosemide therapy.

DOMPERIDONE

Uses: Nausea and vomiting, reflux esophagitis, dyspepsia.

Doses: PO– 0.3 mg/kg/dose q 4–8 hr.

Brands: 10 mg tablet; 1 mg/mL syrup; Domperon, Domstal, Normetic. 1 mg/mL drops; Vomistop.

Combinations:
- Domperidone + PCM: 10 + 500 mg tablet; Dompar, Domstal-P, Motinorm-P
- Domperidone + Pantoprazole: 10 + 20 mg tablet; Dompan
- Domperidone + Ranitidine: 10 + 150 mg tablet; Gaspaz
- Contraindicated in gastrointestinal (GI) obstruction or perforations. May increase prolactin secretion leading to gynecomastia in males and galactorrhea in females.

GRANISETRON

Uses: Antiemetic in chemotherapy, radiation related and postoperated nausea and vomiting.

Dosage:
- IV– children >2 years—10–20 µg/kg ½ hour before chemotherapy; 2–3 doses may be given
- PO– adults—1 mg bd or 2 mg od 1 hour before chemotherapy.

Brands: 1 and 2 mg tablet; 1 mg/mL injection; Granicip, Topit. 1 mg/mL drops; Graniset.
- May cause hypo- or hypertension, arrhythmias, agitation.

MECLIZINE

Uses: Motion sickness, vertigo, nausea, and vomiting.

Dosage: PO– ≥12 years
- Vertigo: 25–100 mg/day in divided doses
- Motion sickness: 25–50 mg 1 hour before journey.

Brands: Available in combination:
- Meclizine 12.5 mg + Nicotinic acid 50 mg: Diligan tablet
- Meclizine 12.5 mg + vitamin B_6 50 mg: PNV tablet.

METOCLOPRAMIDE

Uses: Gastroesophageal reflux, prevention of nausea and vomiting due to various causes, symptomatic treatment of diabetic gastric stasis.

Dosage:
- Gastroesphageal reflux: PO, IV, IM—0.4–0.8 mg/kg/day divided q 6–8 hr
- Postoperative nausea and vomiting: IV—0.1–0.2 mg/kg/dose
- Chemotherapy-induced vomiting: PO, IV—1–2 mg/kg/dose q 2–4 hr as required.

Brands: 100 mg tablet; 5 mg/mL syrup; 5 mg/mL injection; Maxeron, Perinorm, Reglan, etc.

- Contraindicated in gastrointestinal (GI) obstruction, past history of seizures. Causes extrapyramidal reactions and these can be prevented and treated with diphenhydramine.

ONDANSETRON

Use: Prevention of nausea and vomiting of various etiology.

Dosage:
- PO: <4 years 1–3 mg; 4–11 years 4 mg; >11 years 8 mg q 8 hr
- IV: 0.15–0.45 mg/kg/dose q 8 hr.

Brands: 4 and 8 mg tablet; 2 mg/5 mL syrup; 4 mg/mL injection; Emeset, Ondem, Periset.

Administration: For IV dilute to 1 mg/mL and be given over 15 minutes.

PALONOSETRON

Uses: Chemotherapy-induced nausea and vomiting.

Dasage: 1 month–18 years—20 µ/kg slowly over 15 minutes (maximum dose: 1500 µg). Always give ½ hour before chemotherapy.

Brands: 0.25 mg/mL injection; Chepatron, Palnox, Palzen. 0.5 mg tablet; Eme. od.

PROCHLORPERAZINE

Uses: Nausea, vomiting, vertigo, severe intractable migraine.

Dosage: Not indicated in <2 years or <9 kg
- PO: 0.4 mg/kg/day divided q 6–8 hr
- IM: 0.1–0.15 mg/kg/day divided q 8–12 hr.

Brands: 5 mg tablet; Bemetil, Stemetil, Vometil. 12.5 mg/mL injection; Stemetil, Steminol.
- Chances of extrapyramidal reactions are high in children so always use lowest possible dose.

PROMETHAZINE

Uses: Allergic conditions, motion sickness, antiemetic, and sedation.

Dosage: Not indicated below 2 years of age
- Antihistamine: PO—0.1 mg/kg/dose q 6 hr (maximum: 12.5 mg/day)
- Antiemetic: PO, IM, IV—0.25–1 mg/kg/dose q 6 hr (maximum: 25 mg/dose)
- Sedation: PO, IV, IM—0.5-1 mg/kg/dose q 6 hr (maximum: 50 mg/dose)
- Motion sickness: PO—0.5 mg/kg ½ hour before journey, can be repeated after 12 hours as needed.

Brands: 10 and 25 mg tablet; 5 mg/5 mL Elixir; Phenergan, Prometh, Promet. 5 mg/mL injection; Phenergan.
- IM route is preferred, avoid IV use. May cause hypotension in fast IV and hypertension in slow IV use. Children with dehydration are prone to develop dystonic reactions.

TRIFLUOPERAZINE

Uses: Antiemetic, schizophrenia, short-term treatment of anxiety disorders.

Doses: PO
- Vomiting: 3–5 years: 1 mg/day in 3 divided doses. 6–18 years: 4 mg/day in 3 divided doses.
- Schizophrenia: 3–5 years: 1 mg/day in divided doses. 6–12 years: 2–5 mg/day in divided doses. 12–18 years: 5 mg/day in divided doses (maximum: 6 mg/day).
- Severe anxiety disorder: 3–5 years: 1 mg/day. 6–12 years: 4 mg/day. 12–18 years: 4 mg/day (maximum : 6 mg/day).

Brands: 5, 10 mg tab; Neocalm, Trazine, Trinicalm.
- **Chlorpromazine and hydroxyzine also have antiemetic actions.**
- **Dexamethasone and lorazepam are used as adjunctive antiemetic.**

Antiepileptics

chapter 9

These agents are used to decrease the incidence and severity of seizures due to various etiology. Some agents are used parenterally in the immediate treatment of seizures. Patients may require more than one anticonvusant to control seizures on a long-term basis. Some agents are also used to treat neuropathic pain.These acts by depressing abnormal neuronal discharges in the CNS which are causing seizures.They also prevent the spread of seizure activity, depressing motor cortex, raising seizure threshold or altering levels of neurotransmitters depending on the group used.

ADRENOCORTICOTROPIC HORMONE

Uses: Infantile spasms, muscle weakness in myasthenia gravis,west syndrome.

Dosage: IM, SC– infantile spasms: 5–60 units/kg/day for 1 week to 12 months.

Brands: 60 units/mL injection; Acton Prolongatum. 40 and 80 units/mL injection; Corticotropin.
- Prednisolone 2 mg/kg/day is equally efficacious as adrenocorticotropic hormone (ACTH) for infantile spasms. Do not administer live vaccine while on ACTH therapy.

CARBAMAZEPINE

Uses: Prophylaxis of generalized tonic-clonic, partial, mixed partial or generalized seizures; to relieve pain in trigeminal neuralgia or diabetic neuropathy; treatment of bipolar disorders; myotonic muscular dystrophy, mesial temporal lobe epilepsy syndrome, myoclonus due to subacute sclerosing panencephalitis, attention deficit hyperactivity disorder (ADHD).

Dosage: Dosage must be adjusted according to patients response and serum concentrations:
- <6 years: Initial 5 mg/kg/day in 2–4 divided doses; may increase q 5–7 days by 5 mg/kg based on effect (maximum: 35 mg/kg/day).
- >6 years: Initial 10 mg/kg/day in 2–4 divided doses; increase by 5 mg/kg/day at weekly intervals until desired levels are achieved; usual maintenance: 400–800 mg/day.

Brands: 100, 200, 400 mg tablet; Carbatol, Mazetol, Tegrital. 100 mg/5 mL suspension; Mazetol, Tegrital.
- A high-fat meal may increase the rate of absorption and reduce time to peak concentration. Children <12 years, who receive >400 mg/day, may be converted to extended release preparations using the same total daily dosage. Administer with food to decrease gastrointestinal (GI) upset. Observe patient for excessive sedation especially when starting or increasing therapy. It is not effective in absence, myoclonic, akinetic or febrile seizures; exacerbation of certain seizure types have been seen after initiation of therapy in children with mixed seizure disorders.

CLOBAZAM

Uses: Add on therapy for complex partial, generalized clonic and tonic, absence, myoclonic, atonic, akinetic aepilepsy, cluster seizures.

Dosage: PO—0.25–1 mg/kg/day divided twice or thrice daily.

Brands: 5, 10, 20 mg tablet; Cloba, Clozam, Frisium.
- Contraindicated in acute respiratory and hepatic insufficiency, myasthenia gravis, sleep apnea.

CLONAZEPAM

Uses: Alone or add on drug for absence, akinetic, Lennox-Gastaut syndrome, myoclonic, infantile spasms.

Dosage: PO—initial daily dose: 0.01–0.03 mg/kg/day divided 2–3 doses (maximum dose: 0.05mg/kg/day); increase by maximum of 0.5

mg every third day until seizures are controlled or adverse effects seen. Maintenance dose: 0.1–0.2 mg/kg/day divided 3 times/day (maximum dose: 0.2 mg/kg/day).

Brands: 0.25, 0.5, 1 and 2 mg tablet; Clonotril, Lonazep, Melzep.
- Prolonged use may lead to loss of efficacy.

DIAZEPAM

Uses: Status epilepticus, skeletal muscle relaxant in tetanus, general anxiety, febrile seizures, preoperative sedation.

Dosage:
- Status epilepticus:
  - IV: Neonates (not as a first line drug) 0.1–0.3 mg/kg/ dose given over 3–5 minutes, every 15–30 minutes to a maximum total dose of 2 mg
  - Infants and children: 0.05–0.3 mg/kg/dose given over 3–5 minutes, every 15–30 minutes to a maximum total dose of 5–10 mg
  - Rectal: 0.5 mg/kg, then 0.25 mg/kg in 10 minutes if needed.
- Sedation: PO—0.2–0.3 mg/kg (maximum: 10 mg); IM/ IV—0.04–0.3 mg/kg/dose (maximum: 0.6 mg/kg every 8 hourly if required)
- Febrile seizures prophylaxis: PO—0.1 mg/kg/day divided every 8 hourly; initiate therapy at the first sign of fever and continue for 24 hour after fever is gone.
- Neonatal tetanus: 0.5–5 mg/kg/every 2–4 hourly IV along with chlorpromazine.

Brands: 2 mg/5 mL suspension; calmpose. 2, 5, 10 mg tablet; Anxol, Calmpose, Valium. 5 mg/mL injection; Anxol, Valium, Zepose. 2 mg/mL direct 2 rectal diazepam.
- Rapid IV push may cause sudden respiratory depression, apnea or hypotension. Do not exceed 1–2 mg/min for IV push.
- Contraindicated in respiratory disease and myasthenia gravis.

ETHOSUXIMIDE

Uses: Used for absence, myoclonic, and akinetic seizures.

Dosage:
- PO: Children <6 years—initial dose: 15 mg/kg/day in two divided doses (maximum: 250 mg/dose); increase every 4–7 days; maintenance dose: 15–40 mg/kg/day in two divided doses
- Children >6 years—initial dose: 250 mg twice daily; increase by 250 mg/day every 4–7 days (maximum: 1.5 g/day).

Brands: 250 mg capsule; 50 mg/mL suspension; Zorantin.
- Ethosuximide may increase tonic-clonic seizures in mixed seizure disorder. May cause blood dyscrasias.

FOSPHENYTOIN

Uses: Management of generalized status epilepticus; used for prevention and management of seizures responsive to phenytoin.

Dosage: Loading dose is 15–20 mg/kg. May substitute IV or IM for phenytoin maintenance doses.

Brands: 75 mg/mL injection; Fosphen, Fosolin:
- Fosphenytoin sodium 1.5 mg is equivalent to phenytoin sodium 1 mg. Abrupt withdrawl of fosphenytoin may precipitate status epilepticus. Consider the amount of phosphate delivered by fosphenytoin in patients who require phosphate restriction (each 1.5 mg delivers 0.0037 mmol of phosphate). More water soluble than phenytoin.

GABAPENTIN

Uses: Add on therapy for partial and secondary generalized seizures; neuropathic pain; migraine.

Dosage: PO–
- Children 3–12 years: 15–35 mg/kg/day in three divided doses (maximum dose: 50 mg/kg/day). Children >12 years: Start by 300 mg daily; then increase by 300 mg/day to maximum of 900–3,600 mg/day in three divided doses.

Brands: 300 mg, 400 mg tablet; Gabapin, Neurontin.
- Antacids reduce the bioavailability by 20%. May impair ability to perform activities requiring mental alertness.

LAMOTRIGINE

Uses: Add on therapy of partial seizures and generalized seizures of Lennox-Gastaut syndrome.

Dosage:
- PO: Children 2–12 years on valproic acid– 0.15 mg/kg/ day in two divided doses for 2 weeks; then 0.3 mg/kg/day for next 2 weeks; Maintenance dose is 1–5 mg/kg/ day (maximum dose: 200 mg/day).
- Children 2–12 years on enzyme-inducing antiepileptic drugs (AEDs): 0.6 mg/kg/day in two divided doses for 2 weeks, then 1.2 mg/kg/day for next 2 weeks; maintenance dose is 5–15 mg/kg/day (maximum: 400 mg/day).

Brands: 5, 25, 50 and 100 mg tablet; Lamitor.
- Fatal rashes may occur if high initial doses or rapid dosage increment is done. May cause swelling of glands and photosensitivity.

LEVETIRACETAM

Use: Adjunctive therapy in partial, myoclonic and tonic-clonic serizure.

Dosage: PO
- 4–12 years: Start at 10 mg/kg/dose twice daily, can be increased every 2 week by 10 mg/kg upto a maximum dose of 30 mg/kg/dose twice daily.
- >12 years: Start at 10 mg/kg/dose twice daily, can be increased every 2 weeks to maximum of 1,500 mg twice daily.

Brands: 250, 500, 750 mg tablet; Levtam, Levipil. 100 mg/mL solution; Levroxa.
- Do not stop abruptly. May cause drowsiness, fatigue, and aggressive behavior.

LORAZEPAM

Uses: Status epilepticus, anxiety, sedation and add on antiemetic therapy, postanoxic myoclonus.

Dosage:
- Status epilepticus:

- IV: Neonates—0.05–0.2 mg/kg/dose over 2–5 minutes; may repeat in 10–15 minutes.
- Infants and children—0.1 mg/kg/dose over 2–5 minutes; repeat after 10–15 minutes if required in a dose of 0.05 mg/kg.
- Anxiety/sedation:
  - IV: Neonates—0.1–0.4 mg/kg/dose every 4–6 hourly as needed.
  - Infants and children: 0.05–0.1 mg/kg/dose q 4–8 hours.
  - Antiemetic therapy: IV—0.04–0.08 mg/kg/dose every 6 hourly as needed.

Brands: 1, 2 mg tablet; 2 mg/mL injection; Anxilor, Calmese, Lopez.

Administration: IV– do not exceed 0.05 mg/kg over 2–5 minutes or 2 mg/min; dilute with equal volume of compatible diluent.

- Do not use in comatose patient, pre-existing CNS depression, hypotension and narrow angle glaucoma.

MIDAZOLAM

Uses: Status epilepticus, sedation, continuous IV for sedation of intubated and mechanically ventilated patients.

Dosage: IV:
- Neonates: Conscious sedation during mechanical ventilation; continuous infusion: 0.15–0.5 µg/kg/min.
- Infants >2 months and children:
  - Status epilepticus: Loading dose 0.15 mg/kg followed by continuous infusion of 1µg/kg/min
  - Sedation: 0.05–0.2 mg/kg loading dose; may be repeated after 1–2 hour if required or continous infusion of 1–2 µg/kg/min.

Brands: 1 and 5 mg/mL injection; Fulsed, Midosed, Shortal.

Administration: For IV administer at a concentration of 1–5 mg/mL to be given over 2–5 minutes.

- Sodium content of injection is 0.14 mEq/mL. Contraindicated in shock, pre-existing CNS depression.

NITRAZEPAM

Uses: Absence, myoclonic, infantile spasms, insomnia, partial epilepsy.

Dosage: PO– start with 0.2 mg/kg/day then gradually increase up to 1 mg/kg/day as required divided every 12 hour or HS.

Brands: 2.5, 5, 10 mg tablet; Nitravet, Nitravan.

OXCARBAZEPINE

Use: Add on or monotherapy for partial and generalized tonic-clonic seizures.

Dosage: Not recommended in <3 years: PO—children 3–17 years: Initial dose 8–10 mg/kg/day in 2 divided doses (maximum dose: 600 mg/24 hours); increase over 2 week to 30– 45 mg/kg/day as per response.

Brands: 150, 300, and 600 mg tablet; Oxcarb, Oxeptal, Oxrate, etc. 300 mg/5 mL suspension; Selzic.

- Significant hyponatremia may occur with its use.

PARALDEHYDE

Uses: Add on therapy for refractory status epilepticus; and as sedative.

Dosage:
- IM: 0.15 mL/kg/dose; may repeat after 4–6 hours
- PR: 0.3 mL/kg/dose mixed with 3:1 in coconut oil; may repeat after 4–6 hours.

Brands: 1 g/mL injection; Paraldehyde.

Administration: May cause nerve damage during IM use, inject carefully. Drug react with plastic; use glass syringe.

PHENOBARBITAL

Uses: Management of generalized tonic-clonic and partial seizures; neonatal seizures; febrile seizures in children; sedation; may also be used for prevention and treatment of neonatal hyperbilirubinemia and lowering of bilirubin in chronic cholestasis.

Dosage:
- Anticonvulsant: Status epilepticus; loading dose; IV: 15–20 mg/kg in a single or divided doses (in selected patients, be given additional

5 mg/kg/dose every 15–30 minutes until seizure is controlled or a total dose of 30 mg/kg is reached) be prepared to support respiration. Maintenance dose: PO, IV (usually starts 12 hours after loading; 5–6 mg/kg/day in two divided doses
- Sedation—PO: 2 mg/kg 3 times/day
- Hyperbilirubinemia: PO—3–8 mg/kg/day in 2–3 divided doses.

Brands: 30, 60 mg tablet; 200 mg/mL injection; Fenobarb, Gardenal. 20 mg/5 mL syrup; Gardenal.

- Do not give IV faster than 1 mg/kg/min with a maximum of 30 mg/min for infants and children. Abrupt withdrawal may precipitate status epilepticus. Dietary requirements of vitamins D, K, C, B_{12}, folate, and calcium may be increased with long-term use. May adversely affect the cognitive performance of children treated on a long-term basis.

PHENYTOIN

Uses: Management of generalized tonic-clonic, simple partial and complex partial seizures; prevention of seizures following head trauma/neurosurgery; ventricular arrhythmias including those associated with digitalis intoxication; myotonic muscular dystrophy.

Dosage:
- Status epilepticus: IV; loading dose:
  - Neonates: 15–20 mg/kg in a single or divided dose
  - Infants and children: 15–18 mg/kg in a single or divided dose
    Maintenance dose: Start after 12 hour of loading dose: 6–8 mg/kg/day.
  - Anticonvulsant: Infants and children: PO—loading dose: 15–20 mg/kg in three divided doses. Maintenance dose: Same as IV maintenance dose
  - Arrhythmias: Loading dose; IV: 1.25 mg/kg every 5 minutes, may repeat up to total loading dose of 15 mg/kg. Maintenance dose: Oral– 5–10 mg/kg/day in 2–3 divided doses.

Brands: 50, 100 mg tablet; 50 mg/mL injection; Dilantin, Epsolin. 125 mg/5 mL suspension; Dilantin.

Administration:
- Neonates: Do not exceed IV infusion rate of 0.5 mg/kg/min
- Infants, children: Do not exceed IV infusion rate of 1–3 mg/kg/min; maximum rate: 50 mg/minute; IV injections should be followed by NS flushes to avoid local irritation of the vein. Dilute with NS to a concentration of 1–10 mg/mL and start infusion immediately after preparation. Avoid using in central lines.

PRIMIDONE

Uses: Generalized tonic-clonic, complex partial, and simple partial seizures.

Dosage: PO–
- Neonates: 12–20 mg/kg/day divided 8–12 hourly; may start with lower dosage and titrate upward
- Children <8 years: 10–25 mg/kg/day divided 8–12 hourly
- Children >8 years: Initial dose: 125–250 mg/day at bedtime; increase by 125–250 mg/day q 3–7 days (maximum: 2 g/day).

Brands: 250 mg tablet; Mysoline.
- May increase the metabolism of vitamin K and D; dietary requirement of vitamin D, K, B_{12}, folate, and calcium may increase with long-term use.

PYRIDOXINE

Uses: Pyridoxine-dependent seizures in infants.

Dosage:
- Neonates: 10–100 mg/day
- Infants: 50–100 mg/day

Brands: 10,50 mg tablet; Ignavit. 50 mg vial; Pyridox.
- When giving large IV doses, monitor respiratory rate, heart rate, blood pressure (BP), electroencephalogram (EEG).

THIOPENTAL

Uses: Intractable seizures; induction of anesthesia; raised ICT (Intractanial tension).

Dosage: IV
- Seizures: 2–3 mg/kg; repeat as needed in 1mg/kg/dose
- Increased ICT: Children; 1.5–5 mg/kg/dose; repeat as needed
- Induction of anesthesia: 3–4 mg/kg.

Brands: 500 mg and 1 g injection; Anesthal, Pentothal, Pentone.

Administration: For IV maximum concentration allowed is 50 mg/mL to be given over 1 hour. Rapid IV may cause hypotension or decreased cardiac output.
- Use with caution in patients with asthma or pharyngeal infections because cough, laryngospasm or bronchospasms may occur.

TOPIRAMATE

Use: Add on therapy of primary generalized tonic-clonic or partial onset seizures; Lennox-Gastaut syndrome in patients >2 years of age; migraine.

Dosage: PO—children 2–16 years: Initial 1–3 mg/kg/day divided 12 hours; increase q 1–2 weeks by 1–3 mg/kg/day. Maintenance dose is 5–10 mg/kg/day.

Brands: 25, 50 and 100 mg tablet; Nextop, Topamate, Topex:
- Hyperchloremic metabolic acidosis may occur in some patients. Somnolence and fatigue are the most common central nervous system (CNS) adverse effects in children.

VALPROATE SODIUM

Uses: Simple and complex partial seizures, simple and complex generalized seizures, mixed seizures type, Lennox–Gastaut syndrome, West syndrome.

Dosage: PO, IV
- Neonates: Loading dose for refractory seizures is 20 mg/kg followed by 10 mg/kg/dose q 12 hr.
- Children: Initial; 10–15 mg/kg/day in divided doses; increase by 5–10 mg/kg/day at weekly intervals until desired levels are achieved. Maintenance dose: 30–60 mg/kg/day. Total IV dose is equivalent to the total daily oral dose, however, it should be given divided every 6 hourly.

- Status epilepticus: 20 mg/kg loading dose followed by 5 – 10 mg/kg/dose every 8 hourly.

Brands: 200, 300, 500 mg tablet; Epirate, Varparin, Valparin. 100 mg/mL IV infusion; Encorate. 200 mg/5 mL syrup; Valparin, Epilex.

Administration: For IV maximum concentration allowed is 20 mg/min. Syrup can be used as retention enema in 1:1 dilution with water. Higher doses up to 100 mg/kg/day may be required if used along with phenytoin, carbamazepine, etc. Hepatic failure and pancreatitis resulting in death may occur in children <2 years of age.

VIGABATRIN

Use: Partial seizures and infantile spasms.

Dosage: PO– start with 20–40 mg/kg/day; titrate slowly upto 80–150 mg/kg/day in two divided doses.

Brands: 500 mg tablet; Sobril.
- Do eye examination every 3–6 months if on vigabatrin therapy.

ZONISAMIDE

Uses: Add on therapy for partial and tonic clonic seizures, atypical absence, Lennox–Gastaut syndrome, and juvenile myoclonic epilepsy.

Dosage: PO—infants and children—initial 1–2 mg/kg/day in 2 divided doses, increase dose in increments of 0.5–1 mg/kg/day every 2 weeks (maximum: 12 mg/kg/day).

Brands: 25, 50 mg capsule; Zonisep. 25, 100 mg tablet; Zonegram. 50, 100 mg tablet; Zonit, Zonimid.

Antifungals

chapter 10

An antifungal agent is a drug that selectively eliminates fungal pathogens from a host with minimal toxicity to the host. These are either fungicidal or fungistatic and acts by affecting the permeability of the fungal cell membrane or protein synthesis within the fungal cell itself. With the advent of newer and ever more potent chemotherapeutic, immunosuppressive, and antimicrobial regimens, complications due to fungal infection are on the rise; and therefore antifungals are a very impotant drugs now a days.

AMPHOTERICIN-B

Uses: Severe systemic infections and meningitis caused by *Candida, Aspergillus,* and *Mucor* species, etc. Treatment of visceral leishmaniasis. Liposomal amphotericin B is useful in cases refractory to or intolerant to conventional amphotericin-B therapy.

Dosage: Conventional is started in a test dose of 0.1 mg/kg/dose to a maximum of 1 mg infused over 1 hour. If test dose is tolerated then therapeutic dose of 0.4 mg/kg can be given on the same day. The daily dose then can be increased in 0.25 mg/kg increments to a dose of 1.5 mg/kg/day. Liposomal amphotericin can be used in higher doses up to 2.5–5 mg/kg/day.

- Liposomal amphotericin-B: Empiric therapy in systemic fungal infection; 3 mg/kg/day as once daily infusion. Visceral leishmaniasis; day 1–5; 3 mg/kg once, 3 mg/kg once on days 14 and 21.

Brands: 50 mg vial; Amfocare, Ampholip, Fungizone.

Administration: Can be given over 2–3 hours in a concentration of 0.1–0.5 mg/mL.

- May cause hypokalemia, hypomagnesemia, azotemia, muscle and joint pain, neuropathy. Fever, chills, flushing, hypotension, etc. can be avoided by prior medication with Meperidine and Acetaminophen.
- Monitor sodium, potassium, kidney function test (KFT), and live function test (LFT).
- Avoid drug exposure to light. Reduce nephrotoxicity by saline loading before the infusion.

CASPOFUNGIN

Uses: Candidiasis, Aspergilosis.

Dosage: IV—neonates: 2 mg/kg once daily (maximum: 50 mg/day)
Pediatrics: 4 mg/kg once daily.

Brands: 50,70 mg injetion; Caspogin.

CLOTRIMAZOLE

Uses: Oropharyngeal, cutaneous and vulvovaginal candidiasis, superficial mycosis, dermatophytoses.

Dosage:
- Topical: Apply twice or thrice daily:
- Vaginal: Apply applicator full of 1% cream daily at bedtime for 7–10 day or 100–200 mg vaginal tablet for 3–7 days. Avoid in <3 years of age.
- Mouth application: Apply 10–20 drop to buccal mucosa.

Brands: Mouth paint, cream, powder, lotion, spray all 1%; Candid. 100 and 200 mg vaginal tablet; Candid, Triben. 1% ear drop, Clotrin.

FLUCONAZOLE

Uses: Systemic, oropharyngeal, esophageal, and vaginal candidiasis; cryptococcal meningitis. Fungal infection of eyes, *T. cruris*, *T. corporis*, etc.

Dosage: PO; IV
- Systemic candidiasis: 6–12 mg/kg/day for 28 days
- Oropharyngeal, esophageal candidiasis: 6 mg/kg on day 1, then 3 mg/kg/day for 14–21 days
- Cryptococcal meningitis: 12 mg/kg on day 1, then 6 mg/kg/day for 10–12 weeks
- In neonates <14 days, dosages are same except given q 48–72 hr.

Brands: 50, 150 and 200 mg tablet; 2 mg/mL injection; Forcan, Zocon. 0.3% eye drop; Syscan, Zocon. 2% Zocon dusting powder.
- Increases phenytoin levels.

FLUCYTOSINE

Uses: Infection caused by Candida and *Cryptococcus*.

Dosage: PO—neonates: 75 mg/kg/day divided q 8 hourly.
Pediatrics: 50–150 mg/kg/day divided q 8 hourly (maximum: 2 g).

Brands: 250 mg tablet; Ancobon. 500 mg tablet; Ancobon, Cytoflu.

GRISEOFULVIN

Uses: Tinea infection of skin, hair and nails caused by Microsporum, Epidermophyton, Trichophyton.

Dosage: PO—micronized is used in a dosage of 10–15 mg/kg/day in 2–3 divided doses (maximum: 1,000 mg), whereas ultramicronized is used in dosages of 5–10 mg/kg/day (maximum: 500 mg).
- Duration of therapy: *T. corporis*—2–4 weeks; *T. capitis*: 4–6 weeks; *T. pedis*: 4–8 weeks; *T. unguium*: 3–6 months.

Brands: 125, 250 and 500 mg tablet; Dermonorm, Grisovin, Nufulvin.

GENTIAN VIOLET

Use: Mucocutaneous and cutaneous infection caused by *Candida albicans*.

Dosage: Apply solution under the tongue or on lesion after feeding. Apply to lesion with cotton, avoid application over ulcerative lesions of face.

Brands: 1 and 2% Gentian violet solution.

HAMYCIN

Use: Candidal oral thrush.

Dosage: Apply 2–3 times/day for 7–10 days.

Brands: Hamycin suspension 200,000 unit/mL.

ITRACONAZOLE

Use: Active against *Candida, Cryptococcus, Aspergillus* and *Histoplasma*.

Dosage: PO—3–5 mg/kg/day once daily.

Brands: 100 mg capsule; Candistat, Canditral, Itracan.

- Decreased effect occurs with Rifampicin, Carbamazepine, Phenytoin, Omeprazole.

KETOCONAZOLE

Uses: Candidiasis, blastomycosis, histoplasmosis, oral thrush; topically for *T. corporis, T. cruris, T. versicolor* and cutaneous candidiasis. Shampoo is used for dandruff.

Dosage: PO—>2 years of age: 3.3–6.6 mg/kg/day once daily (maximum: 400 mg/day).

Brands: 200 mg tablet; Fungicide, Ketozole, Nizral. 2% shampoo; Danruf, Funginoc, Nizral. 2% solution; Arcolane, Dandoff. 2% ointment; Funginoc, Phytoral.

- Avoid antacids, H_2 blockers within 2 hours of use ketoconazole as gastric acidity is necessary for good absorption of ketoconazole.

MICAFUNGIN

Uses: Candidiasis, Aspergillosis.

Dosage: IV—neonates: 10 mg/kg once daily.
            Children: 2-4 mg/kg once daily.

Brands: 50 mg/vial; Micafung-Plus, Mycomine.

MICONAZOLE

Uses: Vulvovaginal candidiasis, topical treatment of superficial fungal infection.

Dosage: >2 years of age—topically apply twice daily. Vaginal; apply one applicator full of cream at bedtime for 7 days.

Brands: 2% ointment; powder and lotion; Zole. 2% vaginal cream; Gynodactrin.

NYSTATIN

Uses: Mucocutaneous, oral, vaginal fungal infection.

Dosage:
- Neonates: 100,000 units qid.
- Infants: 200,000 units qid
- Children: 400,000–600,000 units qid
- Topically: Apply twice or four times/day.

Brands: 500,000 units tablet; Mycostatin. 100,000 units vaginal tablet; Mycostatin vaginal.

SERTACONAZOLE

Uses: Superficial fungal infection, yeast and dermatophyte fungi.

Dosage: Applied locally twice daily.

Brands: 2% cream; Onobet, Seriva, Sertipose.

TERBINAFINE

Uses: Onchomycosis and ringworm.

Dosage: PO—for <20 kg: 62.5 mg/day once; 20–40 kg: 125 mg/day; >40 kg: 250 mg/day. Topically: Apply twice.

Brands: 125, 250 mg tablet; 1% cream; Exifine, Terbifin.

Duration: Finger nails infection 6 week; toenails 12 weeks and Tinea for 2 weeks.

TOLNAFTATE

Uses: *T. pedis, T. cruris, T. corporis, T. manuum* and *T. versicolor*.

Dosage: Apply 2–3 times/day for 2–4 weeks.

Brands: Cream and solution; Tinaderm, Tinavate.

VORICONAZOLE

Uses: Invasive a spergillosis, esophageal candidiasis, infections caused by *Fusarium, Malassezia*.

Dosage: IV—6 mg/kg/dose q 12 hr for 2 doses followed by 4 mg/kg/dose q 12 hr. PO—3–5 mg/kg/dose q 12 hr.

Brands: 200 mg tablet; 200 mg vial; Voraze.

Administration: Given IV over 1–2 hours at a rate of 3 mg/kg/hour; final concentration should be 0.5–5 mg/mL. Orally should be taken empty stomach.

Antigout Agents

chapter 11

In gout, there occurs excess uric acid in the blood which then forms sharp crystals in and around the joints, causing painfull attacks. Antigout agents are also called as antihyperuricemic agents. These agents either correct overproduction or under excretion of uric acid and also decrease pain and inflammation of acute attacks.

ALLOPURINOL

Uses: To prevent attacks of gouty arthritis and nephropathy; treatment of secondary hyperuricemia during chemotherapy of tumors or leukemia, Duchenne's muscular dystrophy.

Dosage: PO
- ≤10 years: 10 mg/kg/day divided q 8 hr (maximum 400 mg/day).
- >10 years: 200–600 mg/day divided q 8 hr.

Brands: 100 and 300 mg tablet; Aloric, Ciploric, Zyloric.
- Administer with plenty of fluids. May cause rashes, exfoliative dermatitis, leukopenia, thrombocytopenia, hepatitis, peripheral neuropathy. Discontinue drug use at first sign of rash.

COLCHICINE

Uses: Acute and chronic gouty arthritis, Mediterranean fever.

Dosage: PO—acute attack; 0.5–0.6 mg q 2 hr till the pain is relieved or gastrointestinal (GI) toxicity occur (maximum: 8 mg/day).
- Mediterranean fever prophylaxis: <5 years: 0.5 mg/day, >5 years: 1–1.5 mg/day in 2–3 divided doses.

Brands: 0.5 mg tablet; Coljoy, Zycolchin.
- Side effects as of Allopurinol.

PROBENECID

Uses: Prevention of gouty arthritis; also prolongs serum level of penicillin/cephalosporins.

Dosage: PO—initial dose of 25 mg/kg as single dose followed by 40 mg/kg/day divided q 6 hr (maximum single dose: 500 mg).

Brands: 500 mg tablet; Bencid.

- Contraindicated in <2 years of age, blood dyscrasias, uric acid renal stones. Drink plenty of fluids to reduce the risk of uric acid stones.

Anthelmintics

chapter 12

ALBENDAZOLE

Uses: Active parenchymal neurocysticercosis lesions of *Taenia solium;* cystic hydatid disease of liver, lung, and peritoneum caused by *E. granulosus; ascariasis, A. duodenale, Necator americanus, Enterobius, Trichuris trichiura, giardiasis.*

Dosage:
- Neurocysticercosis: 15 mg/kg/day in two divided doses for 28 days (maximum: 800 mg/day)
- Hydatid disease: 15 mg/kg/day in 2 divided doses for 1–6 months (maximum: 800 mg/day)
- Ascariasis, hookworm, whipworm: 400 mg as a single dose in >2 years of age and 200 mg single in <2 years of age
- Cutaneous larva migrans: 400 mg once daily for 3 days
- *Enterobius:* 400 mg as a single dose; repeat in 2 weeks
- Trichinosis: 400 mg twice daily for 8–14 days
- Visceral larva migrans: 400 mg twice daily for 5 days
- Giardiasis: 400 mg once a day for 5 days.

Brands: 400 mg tablet; 200 mg/5 mL syrup; Albendal, Nemazole, Zental.

Combinations: Albendazole + Ivermectin.

Use carefully in impaired hepatic function and decreased total leukocyte count (TLC). Corticosteroids should be administered 1–2 days before initiating albendazole therapy in patients with neurocysticercosis and should be followed by concurrent steroid and anticonvulsant therapy for the first week. Retinal lesions with neurocysticercosis is a contraindication for albendazole therapy. Bioavailability is increased with fatty meal.

DIETHYLCARBAMAZINE (DEC)

Uses: Lymphatic filariasis (*B. malayi, B. timori, Wuchereria bancrofti*), tropical eosinophilia, Loeffler's pneumonia due to ascariasis.

Dosage: Due to dose related complications, dose of DEC should be increased gradually.
- Tropical eosinophilia: 10 mg/kg/day q 8 hr for 1 month
- Loeffler's pneumonia: 15 mg/kg/day single dose for 4 days
- For patients with high microfilaria levels: 1 mg/kg single dose on day 1; 1 mg/kg tid on day 2; 1–2 mg/kg tid on day 3; 6 mg/kg/day tid divided on days 4–14. For patients with no microfilaria in the blood 6 mg/kg/day divided tid for 4–14 days.

Brands: 50, 100 mg tablet; 120 mg/5 mL syrup; Banocide Hetrazan. 50 mg/5 mL syrup; Banocide.

IVERMECTIN

Uses: Ascariasis, enterobiasis, strongyloidosis, filariasis, onchocerciasis, scabies, pediculosis.

Dosage: PO–0.2 mg/kg single dose. May be repeated after 14 days.

Brands: 3,6,12 mg tablet; Ivermectol, Scavita, Vermin.

LEVAMISOLE

Uses: Ascariasis, hookworms, mixed infestations and as immunomodulator.

Dosage: PO
- Ascariasis: 2 mg/kg/day single dose
- Hookworm: 50 mg q 6 hr for four doses
- Immunomodulator: 2 mg/kg/day every alternate day for 1 month.

Brands: 50 and 150 mg tablet; Dewormis, Levomol, Vermisol. 50 mg/5 mL syrup; Vermisol.

MEBENDAZOLE

Uses: Enterobiasis, trichuriasis, ascariasis, hookworm infections.
Dosage: PO
- Pinworms: 100 mg single dose; may need to repeat after 2 weeks

- Whipworms, roundworms, hookworms: 100 mg twice daily for 3 days, if not cured within 3–4 weeks, a second course may be given
- Capillariasis: 200 mg twice a day for 20 days.

Brand: 100 mg tablet; 100 mg/5 mL syrup; Mebex, Wormin, etc.

NICLOSAMIDE

Uses: Treatment of tapeworm infections (beef, fish, dog, and cat).

Dosage: Avoid below 2 years of age:
- Beef and fish tapeworms: 40 mg/kg once (maximum: 2 g)
- Dwarf tapeworms: 40 mg/kg/day for 7 days (maximum: 2 g/day).

Brands: 500 mg tablet; Niclosan, Nicloside.

PIPERAZINE

Uses: Pinworms and roundworms.

Dosage: PO
- Pinworms: 65 mg/kg/day once daily for 7 days
- Roundworms: 75 mg/kg/day once daily for 2 days.

Brands: 750 mg/5 mL syrup, 500 mg tablet; Piperazine citrate, Antepar.
- Incresed risk of abnormal movements with phenothiazines and antipsychotics.

PRAZIQUANTEL

Uses: Schistosomiasis (all stages), many intestinal tapeworms and trematode infections.

Dosage: PO
- Schistosomiasis: 20 mg/kg/dose q 8 hr for 1 day
- Cysticercosis: 50 mg/kg/day q 8 hr for 15 days
- Tapeworm: 5–10 mg/kg single dose.

Brands: 500 mg tablet; Cysticide. 600 mg tablet; Prazine.
- Contraindicated in spinal and ocular cysticercosis. Use steroids prior to starting praziquantel in neurocysticercosis; dexamethasone is recommended for patients with numerous cysts.
- Cimetidine increases, carbamazepine and phenytoin decreses blood level of praziquantel.

PYRANTEL PAMOATE

Uses: Ascariasis, hookworm, pinworm and trichostrongyliasis infections.

Dosage: Contraindicated below 2 years of age:
- Pinworm, roundworm, trichostrongyliasis: 100 mg once; may repeat in 2 weeks
- Hookworms, roundworms, whipworms: 11 mg/kg single dose (maximum dose: 1 g); may repeat in 2 week for pinworm.

Brands: 250 mg tablet; 250 mg/5 mL suspension; Nemocid, Expent.

THIOBENDAZOLE

Uses: Cutaneous larva migrans, guinea worm, trichinosis, hookworm, trichuriasis, strongyloidosis, toxocariasis.

Dosage: PO
- Cutaneous larva migrans, Guinea worm, Strongiloidosis, Trichuriasis, hookworm: 25 mg/kg, 2 times daily for 2 days.
- Trichinosis: 25 mg/kg, 2 times daily for up to 7 days.
- Toxocariasis: 25 mg/kg, 2 times daily for 7 days.

Brands: 500 mg tablet, 500 mg/5 mL suspension; Tiabendazole, Equizole.

Antihistamines

chapter 13

These drugs are used for relief of symptoms associated with allergies including rhinitis, urticaria, angioedema, and as adjunctive therapy in anaphylactic reaction. These acts by blocking the effect of histamine at H1 receptor. Most antihistamines have anticholinergic properties and may cause constipation, dry eyes and mouth, blurred vision. Also causes sedation. Should not be used in premature or newborn infants. Additive sedation seen when used with other CNS depressants (antidepressants, opioid analgesics, and sedative/hypnotics).

ASTEMIZOLE

Uses: Allergic rhinitis and conjunctivitis, chronic allergic dermatological problems, etc.

Dosage: PO–given once daily. <6 years: 0.2 mg/kg; 6–12 years: 5 mg; >12 years: 10–30 mg.

Brands: 10 mg tablet; 5 mg/5 mL syrup; Acemiz, Stemiz.
- Avoid abrupt discontinuation.
- This is now under banned category drug.

AZATADINE

Uses: Allergic rhinitis, allergy, urticaria, etc.

Dosage: PO—1–6 years: 0.25 mg and >6 years: 0.5–2 mg two times/day.

Brands: 0.5 mg/5 mL syrup; 1 mg tablet; Zadine.

AZELASTINE

Uses: Allergic conjunctivitis, allergic rhinitis.

Dosage: Allergic conjunctivitis:(0.05% solution); 4–18 years; Apply 1–2 drops 2 times daily, increase to 4 times if necessary. Rhinitis: >5 years; 140 µg nasal spray in each nostril.

Brands: 0.05% eye drop; Oculast. 0.1% nasal spray; Azelast.

CETIRIZINE

Uses: Allergic rhinitis, chronic idiopathic urticaria, various allergies.

Dosage: PO–avoid below 2 years of age:
- 2–5 years: 2.5 mg/day once or two divided doses
- >6 years: 5–10 mg/day once or two divided doses.

Brands: 10 mg tablet; 5 mg/5 mL syrup; Alerid, Cetiriz, Cetzine, Hicet, Zyrtec.

CHLORPHENIRAMINE MALEATE

Uses: Allergic rhinitis, motion sickness, various allergic symptoms.

Dosage: PO
- 2–5 years: 1 mg q 4–6 hr; 6–11 years: 2 mg q 4–6 hr (maximum: 12 mg)
- >12 years: 4 mg q 4–6 hr (maximum: 24 mg).

Brands: 4 mg tablet; Cadistin, Piriton.
- Available in combination with chlorpheniramine (CPM), phenylephrine, paracetamol (PCM), dextromethorphan in anticold preparations.

CLEMASTINE FUMARATE

Uses: Allergic rhinitis and various allergic symptoms.

Dosage: PO–avoid below 1 year of age.
- 1–6 years: 0.3–0.5 mg/kg/day divided 8–12 hours (maximum: 1 mg)
- 6–12 years: 0.5–1.2 mg/kg/day divided 12 hours (maximum: 2 mg)
- >12 years: 1.3–2.5 mg/kg/day divided 12 hours (maximum: 5 mg).

Brands: 1 mg tablet; 0.5 mg/5 mL syrup; Clamist, Tavegyl.

CYPROHEPTADINE HYDROCHLORIDE

Uses: Various allergic symptoms, appetite stimulant, migraine prophylaxis, beingn paroxysmal vertigo.

Dosage: PO–0.25 mg/kg/day divided 8–12 hours or:
- 2–6 years: 2 mg q 8–12 hr, >6 years: 4 mg q 8–12 hr
- Migraine: 0.2–0.4 mg/kg at bedtime.

Brands: 4 mg tablet; 2 mg/5 mL syrup; Ciplactin, Peritol, Practin.

DESLORATADINE

Uses: Allergic rhinitis, chronic idiopathic urticaria.

Dosage: PO
- 2–5 years: 1.25 mg/day od
- 6–12 years: 2.5 mg/day od
- >12 years: 5 mg/day od.

Brands: 5 mg tablet; Desent, Loreta, Neoloridin.

DIPHENHYDRAMINE

Uses: Allergic symptoms, mild night time sedation, motion sickness, antitussive, phenothiazine-induced dystonic reactions.

Dosage: PO–
- Dystonic reactions and allergic reactions: 5 mg/kg/day divided q 6–8 hr (maximum: 300 mg/day)
- Antitussive: 2–6 years: 6.25 mg; 6–12 years: 12.5 mg; >12 years: 25 mg q 4 hr
- Night time sleep: 2–12 years: 1 mg/kg/dose (maximum dose: 5 mg) >12 years: 50 mg.

Brands: 25 mg capsule; 12.5 mg/5 mL syrup; Benadryl. 12.5 mg tablet; 12.5 mg/5 mL syrup; Cofryl.

EBASTINE

Uses: Allergic rhinitis, chronic idiopathic urticaria.

Dosage: PO: 6-18 years: 5-10 mg once daily without regards to food.

Brands: 5,10,20 mg tab; Best, Ebast, Ebay.

FEXOFENADINE

Uses: Seasonal allergic rhinitis, chronic idiopathic urticaria.

Dosage: PO—6 months to 2 years; 15 mg once daily. 2–6 years: 15 mg twice daily. 6–12 years: 30 mg od, >12 years: 60 mg bd or 180 mg od.

Brands: 30, 60 and 120 mg tablet; 60 mg/5 mL syrup; Altiva. 120 and 80 mg tablet; 30 mg/5 mL syrup; Fexidine.
- Erythromycin and ketoconazole increases fexofenadine plasma levels by decreasing its metabolism.

HYDROXYZINE

Uses: Allergy, anxiety, preoperative sedation and antiemetic.

Dosage: PO—2 mg/kg/day divided q 6–8 hr. IM: 0.5–1 mg/kg/ dose q 4–6 hr.

Brands: 10 mg and 25 mg tablet; 10 mg/5 mL syrup; 6 mg/ mL drops; 25 mg/mL injection; Atarax, Hicope, Hyzer.

KETOTIFEN

Uses: Bronchial asthma, allergic rhinitis, allergic conjunctivitis.

Dosage: PO
- Children >2 years: 1 mg once daily with food.
- Adolescents: 1–2 mg once daily with food.

Brands: 1 mg/5 mL suspension; 1 mg tablet; Asthafen, Ketotif, Ketasma, Zerosma.

LEVOCETRIZINE

Uses: Allergic rhinitis, urticaria.

Dosage: PO—should be given at evening time.
- 2–6 years: 0.125 mg/kg once daily. 6–11 years: 2.5 mg once daily. >12 years: 5 mg once daily.

Brands: 2.5 mg/5 mL suspension; 5 mg tablet; Airitis, Levocet, Laveta, Zipcet.
- Use with caution in epileptic patients and patients at risk of convulsions.

LORATADINE

Uses: Allergic rhinitis, chronic idiopathic urticaria.

Dosage: PO—2–5 years: 5 mg od, >5 years: 10 mg od.

Brands: 10 mg tablet; 5 mg/5 mL syrup; Alaspan, Loridin, Roletra.
- Macrolides, ketoconazole, theophylline decreases its metabolism.

PHENIRAMINE

Uses: Allergic rhinitis, urticaria, pruritus, drug rash.

Dosage: PO, IM, IV: 0.3–0.5 mg/kg/day divided q 8 hr.

Brands: 25 and 50 mg tablet; 22.75 mg/mL injection; Avil.

PROMETHAZINE

Refer Chapter 8 'Antiemetics'.

PSEUDOEPHEDRINE

Uses: Nasal congestion due to common cold, upper respiratory allergies and sinusitis, also helps in sinus and nasal drainage.

Dosage: PO
- <2 years: 4 mg/kg/day divided q 6 hr.
- 2–5 years: 15 mg q 6 hr; maximum: 60 mg/day
- 6–12 years: 30 mg q 6 hr; maximum: 120 mg/day
- >12 years: 60 mg q 6 hr; maximum: 240 mg/day.

Brands: 60 mg tablet; 30 mg/5 mL syrup; Sudafed.

Antihypertensives

chapter 14

These agents are used for the treatment of hypertension (HT) of various causes, most commonly essential hypertension. Parenteral preperations are used in the treatment of hypertensive emergencies. Oral treatment should be initiated as soon as possible and individualized to ensure adherence and compliance for long-term therapy. Therapy is initiated with agents having minimal side effects. When such therapy fails more potent drugs with different side effects and mode of action are added in an effort to control blood pressure (BP) while causing minimal patient discomfort. The goal of therapy is prevention of end organ damage and overall well-being.

AMLODIPINE

Uses: Hypertension

Dosage: PO—>6 years: 100–200 µg/kg once daily; can be increased to maximum of 10 mg (6–15 kg: 1.25 mg, 15–25 kg: 2.5 mg, >25 kg: 5 mg).

Brands: 2.5, 5, 7.5, 10 mg tablet; Amlomg. 2.5, 5, 10 mg tablet; Amlopres, Amcard, Stamlo. 1.25, 2.5, 5 mg tablet; Eslo.

ATENOLOL

Uses: Hypertension, alone or in combination; antiarrhythmic.

Dosage: PO—0.8–1.5 mg/kg/day (maximum: 2 mg/kg and do not exceed 100 mg/day).

Brands: 25, 50 and 100 mg tablet; Aten, Atenova, Betacard, Tenolol.

- Contraindicated in pulmonary edema, cardiogenic shock, bradycardia, heart block, uncompensated congestive heart failure. Discontinue drug over 1–2 weeks and always avoid abrupt withdrawal. May mask signs of hyperthyroidism.

CAPTOPRIL

Uses: Hypertension and CHF.

Dosage: Must be titrated according to patient response PO:
- Neonates: 0.05–0.1 mg/kg/dose q 8–24 hr (maximum: 0.5 mg/kg/day)
- Infants: 0.15–0.3 mg/kg/dose q 8–24 hr (maximum: 6 mg/ kg/day)
- Children: 0.3–0.5 mg/kg/dose q 8–24 hr (maximum: 6 mg/ kg/day).

Brands: 12.5 and 25 mg tablet; Aceten, Capace, Capotril.
- May cause neutropenia, agranulocytosis, cough, angioedema. Long-term use may lead to zinc deficiency
- Food decreases absorption by approximately 50%. Administration time need to be consistent, given at least 1 hour before meals.

CARVEDILOL

Uses: Supraventricular and other tacharrhythmias, HT; mild, moderate or compensated heart failure, secondary to ventricular dysfunction.

Dosage: PO–0.1 mg/kg/day in 2 divided doses, can be increased at 1–2 weekly intervals to 1 mg/kg/day.

Brands: 3.125, 6.25, 12.5, 25 mg tab; Carditone, Carvas, Carvedil.

CLONIDINE

Uses: Hypertension, alternate agent for attention deficit hyperactivity disorder (ADHD), aid in the diagnosis of pheochromocytoma and growth hormone deficiency, migraine prophylaxis, narcotic withdrawl.

Dosage: Children; PO
- Hypertension: 5–10 µg/kg/day divided q 8–12 hr (maximum: 0.9 mg/day)
- ADHD: Start at 0.05 mg/day, increase q 3–7 days by 0.05 mg/day, given divided q 3–4 hr (maximum: 0.4 mg/day)
- Clonidine tolerance test: Test of growth hormone release from pituitary; 4 µg/kg as single dose.

Brands: 100 µg tablet; Arkamin.150 µg tablet; Catapres.150 µg injection; Arkamin, Catapres.

- Abrupt withdrawal may lead to rapid increase in blood pressure and symptoms of sympathetic over activity, so taper gradually over more than a week.

DIAZOXIDE

Uses: Emergency lowering of blood pressure, hypoglycemia related to hyperinsulinism.

Dosage:
- Hypertension: Children; IV: 1–3 mg/kg, may be repeated in 5–15 minutes (maximum: 150 mg/dose)
  Hyperinsulinemic hypoglycemia: PO
- Newborns and infants: 8–15 mg/kg/day divided q 8–12 hr
- Children: 3–8 mg/kg/day divided q 8–12 hr.

Brands: 15 mg tablet; Eudemine. 15 mg/ml inj; Eudemine, Hyperstat.
- If beta blockers, hydralazine, nitrates are already in use in a patient, then use of diazoxide is not recommended within 6 hours.

DILTIAZEM

Uses: Hypertension, atrial fibrillation or flutter, paroxysmal supraventricular tachycardia (PSVT).

Dosage: PO
- Children: 1.5–2 mg/kg/day in 3–4 divided doses.

Brands: 30 and 60 mg tablet; Cardem, Dicard, Dilzam, Masdil.
- Contraindicated in second or third degree heart block, sick sinus syndrome. Should not be stopped abruptly. May lead to bradycardia, hypotension, CHF, hepatic injury.

ENALAPRIL

Uses: Hypertension, CHF.

Dosage: PO
- Neonates: 0.1 mg/kg/day in divided doses (maximum: 0.4 mg/day)
- Infants and children: 0.1–0.5 mg/kg/day in two divided doses.

Brands: 2.5, 5 and 10 mg tablet; Enam, Envas, Minipril, Vasopril.
- Side effects are similar to other angiotensin-converting enzyme (ACE) inhibitors.

HYDRALAZINE

Uses: Hypertension, CHF.

Dosage:
- IM, IV: 0.1–0.2 mg/kg/dose q 4–6 hr (maximum: 3.5 mg/kg/day)
- PO: 0.75–1 mg/kg/day in 2–4 divided doses (maximum: 7.5 mg/kg/day).

Brands: 25 mg tablet and 20 mg/mL injection; Apresoline.
- For IV administration maximum rate permitted is 0.2 mg/kg/min.

LABETALOL

Uses: Hypertension, used IV in hypertensive emergencies.

Dosage:
- PO: 4 mg/kg/day in two divided doses (maximum: 40 mg/day)
- IV: Starting dose 0.2–1 mg/kg/dose (maximum: 20 mg/dose)
  Continuous infusion: 0.4–1 mg/kg/h (maximum: 3 mg/kg/h).

Brands: 10 mg tablet, 5 mg/mL injection; Lobet. 50, 100 and 200 mg capsule; Normadate.
- Contraindicated in asthma, uncomplicated CHF, bradycardia, pulmonary edema.

LISINOPRIL

Use: Hypertension

Dosage: Children >6 years—starting dose is 0.07 mg/kg once daily (maximum: 5 mg/day).

Brands: 2.5, 5, 10 mg tablet; Cipril, Linvas, Zestil.

LOSARTAN POTASSIUM

Uses: HT, chronic CCF.

Dosage: PO—usual dose in children >6 years—0.7 mg/kg once daily (maximum: 50 mg/day).
- Hypertension: Adolescents—initially 50 mg once daily. Maintenance dosage range is 25–100 mg/day.

Brands: 25, 50 mg tablet; Alsartan, Losar, Tozaar, Zaart.

METHYLDOPA

Uses: Hypertension

Dosage: Start at 10 mg/kg/day divided 2–4 hourly, may be increased every 2 days if required to a maximum dose of 65 mg/kg/day.

Brands: 250 mg tablet; Alphadopa, Amdopa, Sembrina.

METOPROLOL

Uses: Hypertension, arrhythmias, idiopathic hypertrophic subaortic stenosis, migraine prophylaxis, cyanotic spells.

Dosage: PO—1–5 mg/kg/day.
- Cyanotic spells: 0.05–0.1 mg/kg over 2 minutes; may be repeated after 5 minutes once.

Brands: 25, 50 and 100 mg tablet; Betaloc, Metolar, Toprol-XL.
- Abrupt discontinuation should be avoided. Contraindicated in sinus bradycardia, CHF, cardiogenic shock.

MINOXIDIL

Uses: Hypertension, topically for alopecia (male pattern).

Dosage:
- Hypertension: PO—start at 0.1–0.2 mg/kg single dose; maximum 5 mg/day; can be increased every 3 day to 0.25–1 mg/kg/day in two divided doses to a maximum of 50 mg/day
- Alopecia: Apply twice daily.

Brands: 2.5, 5 and 10 mg tablet; Loniten. 2% and 5% solution; Coverit, Pilagro, Regrow.
- Minoxidil use should be reserved for patients not responding to maximum dose of diuretics and to other antihypertensive agents. May cause pericarditis, pericardial effusion and tamponade.

NIFEDIPINE

Uses: Hypertension, hypertrophic cardiomyopathy.

Dosage: PO; SL

- Infants and children: 0.25–0.5 mg/kg/dose (maximum: 10 mg/dose or 1–2 mg/kg/day)
- Hypertrophic cardiomyopathy: 0.6–0.9 mg/kg/day in 3–4 divided doses.

Brands: 5 mg capsule, 10 and 20 mg tablet; Angioblock, Cardipin, Depin, Myogard.

- More rapid effect is seen if drug is administered empty stomach. May lead to hypotension, tachycardia, flushing. Concurrent beta blocker use may lead to increase in cardiovascular side effects. Nifedipine increases phenytoin, digoxin, and cyclosporine serum levels.

NITROPRUSSIDE

Uses: Hypertensive crises, CHF, controlled hypotension during anesthesia.

Dosage: IV—initial dose is 0.3–0.5 µg/kg/min, titrate to a desired effect up to maximum dose of 8 µg/kg/min.

Brands: 50 mg/mL injection; Nipress, Pruside, Sonide.

Administration: Dry powder for injection should only be dissolved in 5% dextrose water and should be protected from light. Left over should be discarded after 24 hours of reconstitution. Overdose or prolonged use may lead to cyanide or thiocyanate toxicity.

PHENOXYBENZAMINE

Uses: Symptomatic treatment of sweating and HT in patient with pheochromocytoma.

Dosage: PO—0.2–2 mg/kg/day as single dose.

Brands: Fenoxene 10 mg capsule and 50 mg/mL injection.

- May cause nasal congestion, dizziness, constricted pupils.

PHENTOLAMINE

Uses: Diagnosis and treatment of pheochromocytoma, used locally for extravasation of drugs with alpha adrenergic effects (dopamine, dobutamine, epinephrine, phenylephrine).

Dosage:
- Extravasation: Dilute 2.5–5 mg in 10 mL normal saline and then infiltrate by multiple injections (maximum: 0.1 mg/kg)
- Pheochromocytoma: IM, IV: 0.05–1 mg/kg/dose (maximum: 5 mg).

Brands: Fentanor, Fentosol 10 mg/mL injection.

PRAZOSIN

Uses: Hypertension, severe CHF.

Dosage: PO—0.1 mg/kg/dose q 6 hr, can be increased slowly up to a maximum dose of 0.4 mg/kg/day.

Scorpion envenomation: 0.03 mg/kg/dose, then every 4–6 hourly.

Brands: 2.5 and 5 mg tablet; Minipress, Prazocip XL, Prazopress.
- First dose of a drug may cause marked hypotension, syncope and loss of consoiousness. This effect is more commonly seen in patient of salt or water depletion, receiving beta blocker, diuretics.

PROPRANOLOL

Uses: Hypertension, arrhythmias, tetralogy of Fallot cyanotic spells, migraine prophylaxis, and short-term adjunctive therapy of thyrotoxicosis, essential tremors, portal HT, capillary hemangioma.

Dosage:
- Hypertension, arrhythmias: PO—0.5–1 mg/kg/day divided 6–8 hr, titrated slowly upward up to 2–5 mg/kg/ day. IV: 0.01–0.1 mg/kg/dose to be given over 15 minutes; maximum dose 1 mg in infants and 3 mg in children.
- Migraine prophylaxis: PO—0.6–1.5 mg/kg/day divided q 6–8 hr (maximum: 4 mg/kg/day).
- Tetralogy spells: Starting dose is 1–2 mg/kg/dose every 6 hours, can be titrated upward slowly every 24 hour to maximum of 5 mg/kg/day.
- Thyrotoxicosis: PO—2 mg/kg/day divided q 6–12 hr.
- Arrhythmia/cyanotic spells: PO—2–6 mg/kg/day divided every 6–8 hourly.

Brands: 10, 40 and 80 mg tablet; Ciplar, Inderal. 1 mg/mL injection; Properol.
- Give IV slowly at a rate of 1 mg/min. Taper slowly over 2 weeks. Not indicated in patients with CHF, bradycardia, heart block, asthma. Cimetidine, ciprofloxacin, fluconazole, isoniazid, theophylline may increase propranolol levels and toxicity.

RAMIPRIL

Uses: Hytertension, proteinuria in chronic renal disease.

Dosage: PO—1.5 mg/m^2/day once daily (maximum: 20 mg/day).

Brands: 2.5, 5 mg tablet; Cardace, Hopace, Prilace, Ramipres.

SODIUM NITROPRUSIDE

Uses: Hypertensive crises, systemic HT, acute severe valvular regurgitation, acute heart failure.

Dosage: IV: 0.3–10 µg/kg/min by infusion.

Brands: 50 mg/mL injection; Niside, Nipress, Nitroplus, Pruside.
- Reconstitute 50 mg in 3 mL of D-5%. Then further dilute to a concentration of 50 µg in 1 liter of D-5%. Discard after 24 hour or if solution changes to dark brown or blue. Protect from light. Invasive BP monitoring is recommended when on therapy.

VERAPAMIL

Uses: Hypertension, supraventricular tachyarrhythmias.

Dosage: Not indicated below 2 years of age:
- IV: 0.1–0.2 mg/kg/dose (maximum: 5 mg/dose); second dose can be repeated after 30 minutes if required
- PO: 4–8 mg/kg/day divided q 8 hr.

Brands: 40 mg and 80 mg tablet; Vasopten, Veramil. 25 mg/mL injection, Calaptin, VPL.

Administration: Monitor BP and electrocardiogram (ECG) during IV use. Calcium chloride should be ready to treat hypotension if occurs.

Antileprotics

chapter 15

Hansen disease/leprosy is curable and treated with multidrug therapy (dapsone, clofazamine, rifampsin). Combination therapy is indicated to prevent antimicrobial resistance. The recommended duration of therapy by WHO for paucibacillary tuberculoid (TT) and borderline tuberculoid (BT) disease is 6 months, two drugs (dapsone, rifampsin) given; and for multibacillary lepromatous leprosy (LL), borderline (BB) and borderline lepromatous leprosy (BL) disease is 12 months, three drugs give (dapsone, rifampicin and clofazimine). Alternative agents to treat Hansen disease include minocycline, clarithromycin and some flouroquinolones (levofloxacin, ofloxacin, moxifloxacin). Neuritis must be treated promptly to minimize nerve injury and disability. Treatment with corticosteroids appear to improve nerve function in 2/3 patients. Bone marrow suppression and hepatotoxicity have been reported and should be monitored every 3 months during therapy. After completion of therapy annual follow-up for up to 5 year for paucibacillary, and up to 10 years for multibacillary disease is warranted.

CLOFAZIMINE

Uses: Multibacillary dapsone-sensitive leprosy, lepromatous leprosy, erythema nodosum leprosum, tuberculosis.

Dosage: PO—1 mg/kg/day; maximum 50 mg/day for daily schedule and 4 mg/kg, maximum 300 mg for once monthly doses. Given in combination with dapsone and rifampicin. *Tuberculosis:* 2–3 mg/kg once daily (maximum dose: 200 mg).

Brands: 50 and 100 mg capsule; Clofozine, Hansepran.
- May discolor skin, conjunctiva, tears, sweat. Use with caution in patient with gastrointestinal problems. Increased oto- and nephrotoxicity with other drugs with similar toxicity.

DAPSONE

Uses: Leprosy, dermatitis herpetiformis, prophylaxis against *Pneumocystis carinii* pneumonia as an alternative drug.

Dosage: PO—1–2 mg/kg/day once daily in combination with other agents (maximum: 100 mg/day).

Brands: 25, 50 and 100 mg tablet; Dapsone, Navophone.
- Contraindicated in glucose-6-phosphate dehydrogenase (G6PD) deficiency. May cause hemolysis, leukopenia, cholestatic jaundice, photosensitivity.

RIFAMPICIN

Also *refer* Chapter 21 'Antitubercular'.

Dosage: PO—10–20 mg/kg single dose empty stomach. <50 kg: 450 mg daily, >50 kg: 600 mg daily. Both given in once daily dose.

Antimalarials

chapter 16

Objective of treatment in malaria is to cure infection, prevent morbidity and progression to severe disese; and to prevent emergence of resistance to antimalarials. Complete and successful antimalarial therapy is possible only when the parasite species is known.

THERAPY OF MALARIA

Uncomplicated P. vivax malaria: Chloroquine full course followed by primaquine for 14 days. In chloroquine-resistant areas antimalarial combination therapy (ACT) is used.

Uncomplicated falciparum malaria: ACT for 3 days with single gametocidal dose of primaquine.

Mixed infection (P. vivax + P. falciparum cases): Full course of ACT and primaquine for 14 days.

Severe malaria (Falciparum/vivax): IV Artisunate full course and should be switched to ACT or chloroquine. Primaquine should be given if malaria is vivax.

[ACT: It is the simultaneous use of two or more blood schizontocidal drugs with independent modes of action and thus unrelated biochemical targets in the parasite.]

WHO recommended ACT are:
- Artemether + Lumefantrine
- Artesunate + Amodiaquine
- Artesunate + Mefloquine
- Artesunate + Sulfadoxine + Pyrimethamine

ARTEETHER

Uses: Severe and complicated malaria including cerebral malaria caused by *Plasmodium falciparum*.

Dosage: IM—3 mg/kg/day once daily for 3 days.

Brands: 75 mg/mL injection containing α and β-arteether; E mal, Falcigard, Match, Rapither.

ARTEMETHER

Uses: Severe falciparum malaria, cerebral malaria, multidrug-resistant malaria.

Dosage:
- Severe malaria: IM, PO—3.2 mg/kg loading dose on first day, followed by 1.6 mg/kg daily for 6 days (maximum total: 9.6 mg/kg); this course should be followed by second-line drug for 7 days
- Uncomplicated malaria: PO—4 mg/kg once a day for 3 days plus mefloquine as single dose on second or third day.

Brands: 40 and 80 mg capsule; 80 mg/mL injection; Larither, Malither, Paluther.

ARTEMETHER AND LUMEFANTRINE

Uses: Treatment of *P. falciparum* malaria or mixed infection including *P. falciparum*.

Dosage: PO—artemether and lumefantrine is available in fixed combination ratio of 1:6. Dose can be calculated by artemether content, i.e., 4 mg/kg/day in two divided doses for 3 days. New and recrudescent infection can be treated with a second course.

Brands: 20 + 120/5 mL syrup; 20 + 120 mg, 40 + 240 mg, 80 + 480 mg tablet; Lumerax, Lumart.
- May cause headache, dizziness, myalgia, abdominal pain.

ARTESUNATE

Uses: Severe malaria and chloroquine-resistant falciparum malaria.

Dosage:
- Severe malaria: IM, IV—loading dose of 2.4 mg/kg as a single dose followed by 1.2 mg/kg/dose at 12 and 24 hours, then 1.2 mg/kg/day for

6 days. If patient can take orally shift to oral formulation in a dose of 2 mg/kg/day. This should be followed by second-line drug for 7 days.
- Uncomplicated malaria: PO—4 mg/kg single dose on day 1, followed by 2 mg/kg daily for 4 days plus mefloquine single dose on second or third day.

Brands: 50 mg tablet; 60 mg vial; Falcigo, Falciquine, Ulteria.

Administration: 60 mg dry powder for injection is dissolved in 0.6 mL of 5% sodium bicarbonate, this is then diluted to 3–5 mL with 5% dextrose and give immediately by IV bolus.
- Antagonistic effect is seen if used along with pyrimethamine and sulfonamides.

CHLOROQUINE

Uses: Chemoprophylaxis in sensitive areas, treatment of uncomplicated malaria due to susceptible *Plasmodium* species, extraintestinal amebiasis.

Dosage:
- Acute attack: PO—10 mg base/kg loading dose followed by 5 mg/kg after 6 hours and then at 24 and 48 hours (total dose: 25 mg/kg). IM: 5 mg base/kg (maximum: 200 mg base); may be repeated after 6 hours (maximum: 10 mg/ kg/day).
- Malaria prophylaxis: PO—5 mg base/kg/week on the same day each week; start 1–2 weeks before exposure and continue for 4 weeks after leaving an endemic area (maximum: 300 mg base/week).
- Extraintestinal amebiasis: PO—10 mg base/kg/day single dose for 2–3 weeks (maximum: 300 mg base/day).
- Chikungunya acute stage: 5 mg base/kg/day for a week.
- Juvenile chronic arthritis: 250 mg base daily can be given up to 3 months.

Brands: 250 and 500 mg tablet (base is 150 and 300), 50 mg/5 mL syrup; 40 mg/mL injection; Cloquin, Emquine, Nivaquin-P, Resochin.
- Parenteral dose should not exceed 5 mg base/kg. Use with caution in liver disease, seizure disorder, auditory damage, psoriasis, G6PD deficiency; should not be given empty stomach and in high fever. If vomiting occur within 45 minutes of a dose, that particular dose is to be repeated after taking care of vomiting.

MEFLOQUINE

Uses: Treatment and prophylaxis of falciparum malaria.

Dosage: PO
- Treatment: Loading dose of 15 mg base/kg as single dose followed by 10 mg/kg 8–12 hours later for 1 day (maximum: 500 mg)
- Chemoprophylaxis: 5 mg base/kg weekly (maximum: 250 mg/week). Started 1 week before and continued for 4 week after last exposure.

Brands: 250 mg tablet; Mefax, Meff, Mefque.
- May cause anxiety, hallucination, bradycardia, sinus arrhythmias.

PRIMAQUINE

Uses: Radical cure and prevention of relapse in vivax and ovale malaria. In case of falciparum it may be given for terminal prophylaxis.

Dosage: PO—radical cure; for vivax and ovale only. 0.3 mg base/kg/day for 14 days as single daily dose; after an adequate course of chloroquine (maximum: 15 mg). Terminal prophylaxis/gametocytocidal action in falciparum—0.7 mg of base/kg as single dose.

Brands: 2.5, 7.5 and 15 mg tablet; Leoprime, Malarid.
- Use with caution in G6PD deficiency, in cases of borderline deficiency once weekly dose of 0.6–0.8 mg/kg is given for 6 weeks. Should not be given along with other drugs causing hematological disorders, e.g., chloromycetin, sulfadoxine + pyrimethamine.

PYRIMETHAMINE AND SULFADOXINE

Uses: Prophylaxis and treatment of malaria.

Dosage: PO
- Acute attack: 1 mg/kg of pyrimethamine (PM) or 20 mg/kg of sulfadoxine (SD) as single dose on last day of quinine therapy.
- Malaria prophylaxis: Not recommended due to side effects. Started 2 weeks before entering the endemic area, where chloroquine-resistant falciparum exists.
    - 2–12 months: 1/4 tablet
    - 1–3 years: 1/2 tablet

- 4–8 years: 1 tablet
- 9–14 years: 2 tablet
- >14 years: 3 tablet.

Brands: PM 25 mg + SD 500 mg tablet and PM 12.5 mg + SD 250 mg/5 mL suspension; Pyralfin, Reziz.

- Use with precautions in folate deficiency, asthma, seizure disorder, G6PD deficiency. Contraindicated in megaloblastic anemia, renal insufficiency, <2 months of age. Folic acid supplements should be delayed for 1 week after PM and SD treatment to avoid inhibitory effect on antimalarial efficacy.

QUININE

Uses: Chloroquine-resistant falciparum malaria, severe complicated falciparum malaria.

Dosage: PO—as quinine sulfate: 30 mg/kg/day divided q 8 hr for 7 days. IV, as quinine dihydrochloride: 20 mg/kg loading dose over 4 hours, then 10 mg/kg over 4 hours; every 8 hourly, until can be given orally, for 7–10 days (maximum: 1,800 mg/day). Quinine should always be used in combination with second-line antimalarial drugs. For example:

- Tetracycline: 5 mg/kg q 6 hr for 7days
- Clindamycin: 20–40 mg/kg/day divided q 8 hr for 5 days
- Doxycycline: 3 mg/kg twice a day for 7 days
- Pyrimethamine + sulfadoxine: 1 mg/kg of pyrimethamine or 20 mg/kg of sulfadoxine.
- Tetracycline and doxycycline are not indicated in <8 years of age. Single dose of primaquine is given at the end of therapy as quinine is not effective against gametocytes of falciparum.

Brands: 150 mg/5 mL suspension; 100, 300 and 600 mg tablet; 300 mg/mL injection; Cinkona, QST, Quinarsol.

Administration: IV dose should be given diluted in 5–10% dextrose in a concentration of 1 mg/mL. 12 mg of dihydrochloride salt is equivalent to 10 mg base, maintenance dose is started after 12 hours of loading dose.

- May cause cinchonism, hypoglycemia, hypotension.

OTHER DRUGS USED AS ANTIMALARIALS

These should not be used as single drugs.

CLINDAMYCIN

Uses: Treatment and prevention of malaria.

Dosage: PO—20 mg/kg/day divided q 12 hourly. For 7 days.

Brands: 300 mg tablet; Stofen. 300 mg capsule; Dalcin. Stofin.
Note: Should be given with food and plenty of water.

DOXYCYCLINE

Uses: Treatment and prevention of malaria.

Dosage: PO—treatment: 3.5 mg/kg divided q 12 hourly for 7 days. Prophylaxis: 1.5 mg/kg/day, started 1 week before departure and continued for 4 weeks.

Brands: 100 mg tablet; Doxt, Doxyplus, Megdox.

Antimyasthenics

chapter 17

EDROPHONIUM

Uses: Diagnosis of myasthenia gravis, nondepolarizing muscular blockade antagonist.

Dosage: IV
- Infants: Initial dose of 0.1 mg, if no response then followed by 0.4 mg, total dose is 0.5 mg
- Children: 0.04 mg/kg given over 1 minute, if no response within 45 seconds then followed by 0.16 mg/kg (maximum: 10 mg total).

Brands: 10 mg ampule; Tensilon.

May cause arrhythmias, hypotension, seizures, drowsiness, laryngospasm, bronchospasm, diaphoresis. Keep atropine ready for treatment of cholinergic crises resulting from overdoses.

NEOSTIGMINE

Uses: Treatment of myasthenia gravis, reversal of nondepolarizing neuromuscular blocking agents.

Dosage:
- Myasthenia gravis:
  - Diagnosis: IM, 0.025–0.04 mg/kg as a single dose
  - Treatment: IM, SC: 0.01–0.04 mg/kg q 2–4 hr and oral dose is 2 mg/kg/day q 3–4 hr (maximum: 375 mg/day).
- Reversal of nondepolarizing neuromuscular blockade: 0.025–0.1 mg/kg/dose (total dose: 5 mg). Use in conjunction with atropine or glycopyrrolate.

Brands: 15 mg tablet; Prostigmin, Tilstigmin. 0.5 mg injection; Myostigmin, Prostigmin.

- Does not antagonize succinylcholine. Use with caution in patients of epilepsy, bradycardia, hypothyroidism, asthma.
- When used in conscious child with myasthenia gravis, may cause severe gastrointestinal pain.

PYRIDOSTIGMINE

Uses: Treatment of myasthenia gravis, reversal of neuromuscular blocking agents.

Dosage:
- Infants of myasthenic mother: 0.05–0.15 mg/kg/dose. Titrate dose to desired response.
- Myasthenia gravis: In children 7 mg/kg/day in 5–6 divided doses.
- Reversal of nondepolarizing neuromuscular blockade: 0.1–0.25 mg/kg/dose preceded by atropine or glycopyrrolate.

Brands: 30 and 60 mg tablet, Myestin.

- May cause seizures, headache, bradycardia, salivation, miosis, urinary frequency.
- In newborn infants give 30 minutes to 1 hour before feeds.

Antiprotozoals

chapter 18

AMPHOTERICIN B
Refer Chapter 10 'Antifungals'.

CHLOROQUINE
Refer Chapter 16 'Antimalarials'.

DILOXANIDE FUROATE

Uses: Amibiasis, Amoebic carrier.

Dosage: PO—2–12 years: 20 mg/kg/day. 12–18 years: 1.5 g in 3 divided doses.

Brands: 500 mg tablet; Amiciline, Furamide.

METRONIDAZOLE

Uses: Amebiasis, giardiasis, trichomoniasis, skin and soft tissue infection (SSTI), central nervous system (CNS) infection, intra-abdominal infection, systemic anaerobic infections.

Dosage:
- Amebiasis: PO—35–50 mg/kg/day divided q 8 hr for 10 days
- Other parasites: PO—15–30 mg/kg/day divided q 8 hr
- Anaerobic infection: PO, IV—30 mg/kg/day divided q 6 hr (maximum: 4 g/day).

Brands: 200 and 400 mg tablet; 200 mg/5 mL suspension; Aristogyl, Flagyl, Metrogyl. 5 mg/mL infusion; Flagyl, Metron.

NITAZOXANIDE

Uses: Amebiasis, giardiasis, helminth infections.

Dosage: PO—1–4 years: 100 mg BD; 4–10 years: 200 mg BD; >10 years: 500 mg BD for 3 days.

Brands: 200 and 500 mg tablet; 100 mg/5 mL syrup; Nitacure, Nizonide, Nixide.

- Avoid in <1 year. May cause increase in serum glutamic pyruvic transaminase (SGPT) and creatinine, dizziness, discolored urine, and pale yellow eyes.

ORNIDAZOLE

Uses: Acute intestinal and extraintestinal amebiasis, giardiasis, anaerobic infections.

Dosage: PO—40 mg/kg once a day; 3 days for amebiasis and 2 days for giardiasis.

Brands: 500 mg tablet; 125 mg/5 mL suspension; 5 mg/mL infusion; Dazolic, Ornida.

PAROMOMYCIN SULFATE

Uses: Acute and chronic intestinal amebiasis and asymptomatic cyst passers, balantidiasis, tapeworm infection, giardiasis, cryptosporidiosis, hepatic encephalopathy, visceral leishmaniasis.

Dosage: PO
- Amebiasis: 25–35 mg/kg daily in 3 divided doses for 5–10 days.
- Tapeworm: 11 mg/kg every 15 minutes for 4 doses.
- Giardiasis: 25–35 mg/kg daily in 3 divided dose for 7 days.
- Visceral leishmaniasis: 11–20 mg/kg daily for 10–21 days.

Brands: 250 mg capsule; Humatin.

PENTAMIDINE

Uses: Visceral leishmanias is *P. carinii* pneumonia prevention and treatment.

Dosage: IV, IM
- *P. carinii* pneumonia treatment: 4 mg/kg/day od for 14 days and for prophylaxis 4 mg/kg/dose q 2–4 weeks
- Leishmaniasis: 2–4 mg/kg/day od for 15 days.

Brands: 300 mg vial; Pentacarinate, Pentam.
- Vancomycin, aminoglycoside and amphotericin B may cause additive toxicity. Give IV slowly over a period of 1 hour in a concentration of 6 mg/mL.

SECNIDAZOLE

Uses: Amebiasis and giardiasis.

Dosage: 30 mg/kg single dose (maximum: 2 g).

Brands: 500 mg and 1 g tablet; Ambiform, Etisec, Secnil, Seczol.

SODIUM STIBOGLUCONATE

Use: Leishmaniasis.

Dosage: IV, IM—20 mg/kg/day for 20 days in localized cutaneous leishmaniasis (LCL) and diffuse cutaneous leishmaniasis (DCL) and 28 days for mucosal leishmaniasis (ML) and visceral leishmaniasis (VL). Repeated courses may be required in patients with severe cutaneous lesions, ML or VL cases.

Brands: 100 mg injection; Sodium Stibogluconate.
- May cause myalgias, arthralgias, abdominal discomfort, elevated liver enzymes and hematologic changes.

TINIDAZOLE

Uses: Giardiasis and amebiasis.

Dosage:
- Amebiasis: 60 mg/kg/day single dose for 3 days
- Giardiasis: 50 mg/kg single dose once.

Brands: 300 and 500 mg tablet; Fasigyn, Tini, Tiniba. 150 mg/5 mL suspension; Tini.
- May cause metallic taste, dark urine, neuropathy, seizures, leukopenia.

Anxiolytics/ Sedatives/ Antipsychotics

chapter 19

ATOMOXETIN

Uses: Non-stimulant drug for attention deficit hyperactivity disorder (ADHD).

Dosage: PO—children >6 years and adolescents: Starting dose is 0.5 mg/kg/day can be increased after 3 days to a dose of 1.2 mg/kg/day in 2 divided doses (maximum dose: 100 mg/day).

Brands: 10, 18, 25, 40 mg tablet; Attentrol, Axepta, Tomoxetin.

CHLORDIAZEPOXIDE

Uses: Anxiety, preanesthetic medication, behavioral disorders, emotional disturbances.

Dosage: PO—0.3–0.5 mg/kg/day in divided doses.

Brands: 10 and 25 mg tablet; Dibrium, Librium.
- May cause drowsiness, dizziness, drug dependence.

CHLORPROMAZINE

Uses: Nausea and vomiting, mania, behavioral problems, neonatal tetanus, to relieve restlessness, and apprehension prior to surgery.

Dosage: PO, IM, IV—0.5–1 mg/kg/dose q 6–8 hr. In neonatal tetanus more frequent dosing can be used (every 2 hourly).

Brands: 25, 50 and 100 mg tablet; 25 mg/mL injection; Megatil, Chlorpromazine.
- May cause hypotension with IV use, tachycardia, extrapyramidal reactions, rash, dry mouth, constipation.

CLONIDINE

Uses: Hyperactivity, Tourette syndrome, sedation.

Dosage: PO
- Hyperactivity and Tourette syndrome: 0.05 mg once daily can be increased weekly by 0.05 mg to maximum of 0.4 mg/kg/day in divided doses.
- Sedation: 1 µg/kg/day in divided doses.

Brands: 100 µg tablet; Arkamin, Catapres, Hyperdine.

HALOPERIDOL

Uses: Psychosis, severe behavioral problems, sedation, choreiform movements.

Dosage:
- 3–12 years: PO—initial dose of 0.025–0.05 mg/day given in divided doses, can be increased by 0.25–0.5 mg every week to maximum of 0.15 mg/kg/day
- 6–12 years: IM—1–3 mg/dose q 6–8 hr (maximum: 0.15 mg/ kg/day).

Brands: 0.25, 1.5 and 5 mg tablet; Depidol, Haldol, Serenace. 50 mg/mL injection; Depidol-LA.
- May cause tachycardia, hypo- and hypertension, sweating, extrapyramidal reactions, bronchospasm, seizures, visual disturbances, leukopenia, anemia.

MELATONIN

Uses: Sleep disorders in children with visual impairment, learning disability, cerebral palsy, and autism.

Dosage: PO—2–3 mg ½ hour before sleep. May be increased to 4–6 mg if benefit is not seen in 1–2 weeks.

Brands: 3 mg tablet; Meloset. 10 mg tablet; Zytonin.

METHYLPHENIDATE

Uses: Attention deficit hyperactivity syndrome, narcolepsy, autism spectrum disorder with ADHD.

Dosage: PO—>6 years: 5 mg/dose; 1–2 times/day. Increase at weekly increments of 5 mg/day if required to maximum of 60 mg/day.

Brands: 10 mg tablet; Addwize. 18 mg SR tablet; Addwize. 10, 36, 54 mg tablet; Concerta.

- Avoid giving doses at bedtime, give ½ hour before breakfast and lunch.

OLANZEPINE

Uses: Schizophrenia, mania.

Dosage: PO—12–18 years; 5–20 mg once daily.

Brands: 2.5, 5, 7.5, 10 mg tablet; Manza, Oliza, Opin.

PIMOZIDE

Uses: Schizophrenia, tic disorders, tourette syndrome.

Dosage: PO—schizophrenia: 12–18 years; 1–20 mg/day in 2 divided doses. Tourette syndrome: 2–12 years; 1–4 mg/day in 2 divided doses. 12–18 years; 2–10 mg/day in 2 divided doses.

Brands: 2, 4 mg tablet; Mocep, Neurop. 10 mg tablet; Orap.

- Do annual electrocardiogram (ECG) to monitor QT interval.

RISPERIDONE

Uses: Schizophrenia, ADHD, aggressive behavior, tourette syndrome.

Dosage: 0.5–2 mg once or in 2 divided doses.

Brands: 1 mg/5 mL syrup; 0.5, 1, 2, 4 mg tablet; Risperdal, Risdone, Sizodone.

THIORIDAZINE

Uses: Psychotic disorders, depressive neurosis, behavioral problems.

Dosage: PO—0.5–3 mg/kg/day divided q 8 hr.

Brands: 10, 25 and 50 mg tablet; Delnil, Ridazin, Thioril.

- Use with caution in patients of cardiovascular problems and seizures.

TRICLOFOS

Uses: Insomnia, as sedative in convulsions, recurrent colic.

Dosage: PO—20 mg/kg/dose.

Brands: 500 mg/5 mL syrup; Pedicloryl, Pedicalm.
- May cause rash, nausea, gastrointestinal (GI) disturbances.

TRIFLUOPERAZINE

Uses: Hallucination, delusions, schizophrenia.

Dosage: PO—in 6–12 years of age group. 1 mg/day in two divided doses can be increased gradually to required effect (maximum: 15 mg/day).

Brands: 1 and 5 mg tablet; Schizonil, Trinicalm. 5 and 10 mg tablet; Neocalm, Trazine.
- May cause hypotension, arrhythmias, dystonias, constipation, dry mouth.

Antiretrovirals

chapter 20

The aims of treatment with antiretroviral (ARV) drugs in HIV infected children are to achieve and sustain full human immunodeficiency virus (HIV) ribonucleic acid (RNA) viral load (VL) suppression and minimize short- and long-term ARV drug toxicity. At the time of antiretroviral therapy (ART) initiation, CD4 count and plasma VL should be monitored to establish a baseline to monitor ART benefit. Triple combination therapy is recommended for treating all HIV infected children. ART does not cure HIV infection and therefore require lifelong therapy. ART should be initiated in everyone living with HIV infection at any CD4 cell count and regardless of WHO clinical staging. Within 1 month of starting effective ART in children, plasma HIV RNA VL decrease subsequently and the CD4 count starts to rise. When treating TB patients living with HIV, TB treatment should be initiated first, followed by ART as soon as possible, i.e, within 2–8 weeks.

NUCLEOSIDE/NUCLEOTIDE REVERSE TRANSCRIPTASE INHIBITORS (NRTI)

These acts by inhibiting reverse transcriptase enzyme. They have activity against both HIV-1 and HIV-2. Dual NRTI is the backbone of current combination of various ARV therapies.

Common side effects are nausea, vomiting, rash, discoloration, fever, anorexia, diarrhea, headache, bone marrow suppression. Less common side effect are hypersensitivity, lactic acidosis, hepatic steatosis, pancreatitis, peripheral neuropathy, retinal depigmentation.

ABACAVIR

Dosage: PO
- Children >3 months and <50 kg: 8 mg/kg q 12 hr
- Children >50 kg: 20 mg/kg q 12 hr (maximum: 300 mg/dose).

Brands: 300 mg tablet; Abamune, Abavir.

DIDANOSINE

Dosage: PO
- Children 2 weeks to 8 months: 50–100 mg/m^2/day divided q 12 hr
- 8 months to 13 years: 120 mg/m^2/day divided q 12 hr
- >13 years: 125 mg BD.

Brands: 25, 50 and 100 mg tablet; Dinex. 250 mg capsule; Dinex, Virosine DR.
- Food decreases bioavailability, antacidss and gastric acid antagonist may increase bioavailability.

LAMIVUDINE

Dosage: PO
- Neonates <30 days: 2 mg/kg/dose twice daily
- Infants and children: 4 mg/kg/dose twice daily (maximum: 300 mg/day).

Brands: 150 and 300 mg tablet; Heptavir, Lamuvid. 50 mg/5 mL syrup; Lamivir.

Combinations:
- Lamivudine + Stavudine: 150 + 30 and 150 + 40 mg tablet; Lamistar
- Lamivudine + Zidovudine: 150 + 300 mg tablet; Combivir. Combination with zidovudine prevent its resistance.

STAVUDINE

Dosage: PO—<30 kg; 2 mg/kg/day divided q 12 hr. 30–60 kg: 30 mg twice daily.

Brands: 30 mg and 40 mg tablet; Virostav. 30 mg and 40 mg capsule Stag, Stavir.

- Combination with zidovudine should not be used as it antagonizes the effect.

ZIDOVUDINE

Dosage: PO
- Prophylaxis: Premature infants—4 mg/kg/day divided q 12 hr for up to 4 weeks, then q 8 hr. Term neonates; 8 mg/kg/day divided q 6 hr
- Treatment: Children 6 weeks to 12 years; 480 mg/m^2/day divided q 8 hr. Adolescents; 200 mg thrice daily.

NON-NUCLEOSIDE REVERSE TRANSCRIPTASE INHIBITORS

EFAVIRENZ

Dosage: PO—children >3 years; 10–15 kg: 200 mg; 15–20 kg: 250 mg; 20–25 kg: 300 mg; 25–32.5 kg: 350 mg; 32.5–40 kg: 400 mg; >40 kg: 600 mg; given once daily.

Brands: 200 mg tablet; Viranz. 200 and 600 mg capsule; Efavir, Efferven.

NEVIRAPINE

Dosage: PO
- Neonates: 240 mg/m^2/day once daily for 14 days, then same dose divided q 12 hr for next 14 days, followed by 400 mg/m^2/day divided q 12 hr
- Children: 4 mg/kg once daily for 14 days (maximum: 400 mg/day).

Brands: 200 mg tablet; Neve, Nevimune. 50 mg/5 mL syrup; Nevimune. Should not be given with fattyfoods.

PROTEASE INHIBITORS

Protease inhibitors may cause hyperglycemia, hyperlipidemia, lipodystrophy, increases bleeding tendency, increase in liver enzymes, bone marrow suppression, nephritis, nephrolithiasis, hepatitis, etc.

AMPRENAVIR

Dosage: PO—children 4–16 years and weight <50 kg: 22.5 mg/kg BD.

INDINAVIR

Dosage: PO—1,500 mg/m^2/day divided q 8 hr.

Brands: 400 mg tablet; Virodin. 400 mg capsule; Indivan, Indivir.
- Avoid fatty meals, drink plenty of fluid daily to resolve drug-induced renal colic due to nephrolithiasis.

LOPINAVIR

Dosage: PO—<40 kg: 40 mg/kg/day divided q 12 hr .>40 kg: 800 mg/day divided q 12 hr.

Brands: Lopnavir + Ritonavir: 133.3 mg + 33.3 mg capsule; Lupimune, Ritomax-L.

NELFINAVIR

Dosage: PO (investigational)
- Neonates and children <2 years: 30 mg/kg/day divided q 8 hr
- Children 2–13 years: 60–100 mg/kg/day divided q 8 hr. Administer with meal to optimize absorption.

Brands: 250 mg tablet; Nel, Nelfin.

RITONAVIR

Dosage: PO—400 mg/m^2/daydivided q 12 hr; titrate upward in 50 mg/m^2/dose increment to 800 mg/m^2/day divided q 12 hr.

Brands: 100 mg capsule; Ritomax, Ritomune.
- Adminster with food.

Antitubercular

chapter 21

Children are not only at higher risk of developing the disease but also are more likely to develop the severe form of the disease. So, timely identification and treatment of infectious case in community will reduce the burden of childhood tuberculosis. In pediatric population, only daily dosages of antitubercular drugs are recommended, thrice weekly regimen is no longer recommended.

Types of antitubercular drugs are:
- Drugs with sterilizing activity: It is the ability of the drug to kill all the bacilli in tubercular lesion as rapidly as possible, e.g., rifampicin pyrazinamide.
- Drugs with early bactericidal activity: It is the ability of the drug to kill the dividing mycobacteria, e.g., isoniazid (INH), rifampicin.
- Drugs with resistance prevention activity: These drugs when combined with other drugs can prevent the emergence of resistant mutants to the companion drug, e.g., INH and rifampicin, ethambutol and INH.

CYCLOSERINE

Uses: Adjunctive treatment in pulmonary and extrapulmonary tuberculosis (TB).

Dosage: PO—10–20 mg/kg/day divided q 12 hr (maximum dose: 1,000 mg/day).

Brands: 250 mg capsule; Coxerin, Cyclorine, Myser.
- Contraindicated in epilepsy, depression, anxiety, confusion. May increase daily requirement of vitamin B_{12} and folic acid. Concomitant use of pyridoxine may prevent neurotoxic effects.

ETHAMBUTOL

Uses: *M. tuberculosis* and other mycobacterial diseases.

Dosage: PO—15–20 mg/kg/day once daily (maximum: 1,000 mg/day).

Brands: 200, 400 and 800 mg tablet; Albutol, Combutol, Mycobutol, Themibutol.

- May cause optic and retrobulbar neuritis, hepatotoxicity. Those children whose visual acuity can be determined accurately should be given ethambutol.

ETHIONAMIDE

Uses: *M. tuberculosis* and other mycobacterial diseases.

Dosage: PO—15–20 mg/kg/day once daily (maximum: 1,000 mg/ day).

Brands: 250 mg tablet; Ethide, Ethomid, Myobit.

- May cause hepatotoxicity, peripheral neuropathy, tremor and optic neuritis. If used along with cycloserine and isoniazid may increase nervous system adverse effects. Administer with pyridoxine to prevent neurotoxic effects.

ISONIAZID

Uses: *M. tuberculosis.*

Dosage: PO—5–10 mg/kg/day once daily (maximum: 300 mg/ day).

Brands: 100 and 300 mg tablet; Isonex, Solonex. 100 mg/5 mL suspension; Siozide.

- May cause hepatitis, peripheral neuropathy, dizziness, seizures. Administer 1 hour before or 2 hour after meals. Advice patients to report prodromal symptoms of hepatitis, tingling or numbness of extremities.

PARA-AMINOSALICYLIC ACID

Uses: *M. tuberculosis.*

Dosage: PO—200–300 mg/kg/day divided q 8 hr (maximum: 12 g/day).

Brands: 1 g tablet; Monospas. 4 g sachet; PAS.

- May cause hepatitis, hypokalemia, leukopenia and goitrous hypothyroidism.

PYRAZINAMIDE

Uses: *M. tuberculosis.*

Dosage: PO—30–35 mg/kg/day once daily (maximum: 1,000 mg/day).

Brands: 500, 750 and 1,000 mg tablet; Cavizide, Pyzina, Pza Ciba. 250 mg/5 mL syrup; Pza Ciba.

- May cause arthralgia, hepatotoxicity, gout.

RIFAMPICIN

Uses: *M. tuberculosis*; meningococcal and *H. influenzae* prophylaxis.

Dosage: PO

- Tuberculosis: 10 mg/kg/day empty stomach single dose
- Meningococcal prophylaxis: In neonates, 10 mg/kg/ day divided q 12 hr; in infants and children 20 mg/kg/day divided q 12 hr for 2 days
- *H. influenzae* prophylaxis: In neonates, 10 mg/kg/day once daily and in infants and children, 20 mg/kg/day once daily for 4 days.

Brands: 150, 300, and 450 mg capsule; R-cin, Rimactane, Ticin. 100 mg/5 mL suspension; Rcin, Rimactane, Rimpin.

- May cause hepatotoxicity, gastritis, flu-like illness. May discolor urine, sweat, tears and other body fluid to red-orange color.

Drugs Used for Multidrug-resitant Tuberculosis

For more details also see under respective section.

AMIKACIN

Dosage: IV—20 mg/kg/day once daily (maximum: 1 g).

Brands: 100, 250, 500 mg injection; Amexel, Amidox, Amikef.

BEDAQUILINE

Dosage: For children above 12 years and >33 kg—400 mg daily for 2 weeks and then 200 mg thrice weekly for 22 weeks.

CAPREOMYCIN

Dosage: IM– 15 mg/kg/day once daily (maximum: 1 g).

Brands: 500 mg vial; Capreo, Kopacin.

CLARITHROMYCIN

Dosage: PO—15 mg/kg/day in 2 divided doses (maximum: 500 mg)

Brands: 125 mg/5 mL suspension; 125, 250 mg tablet; Clarinix, Crixan, Synclar.

CLOFAZIMINE

Dosage: PO—2–5 mg/kg/day once daily (maximum: 100 mg)

Brands: 50, 100 mg capsule; Clofaz, Hansepran.

CYCLOSERINE

Dosage: PO—15 mg/kg/day (maximum: 750 mg)

Brands: 250 mg capsule; Myser, Cyclorin.

DELAMANID

Dosage:
- <7 kg: 1.5–2 mg/kg in 2 divided doses.
- 7–23 kg: 25 mg twice daily.
- 24–34 kg: 50 mg twice daily.
- 35 kg: 100 mg twice daily.

KANAMYCIN

Dosage: IM—15–20 mg/kg/day once daily (maximum: 1 g).

Brands: 500, 1,000 mg vial; Kancin, Kanamac.

LEVOFLOXACIN

Dosage: PO—15–20 mg/kg/day once daily (maximum: 1 g).

Brands: 250, 500, 750 mg tablet; 500 mg infusion; Diolaf, Glevo, Levoflox.

LINEZOLID

Dosage: PO/IV—10 mg/kg/day once daily (maximum: 100 mg).

Brands: 600 tablet and injection; Linobid, Walibur.

MOXIFLOXACIN

Dosage: PO/IV—10–15 mg/kg day once daily (maximum: 600 mg).

Brands: 400 mg tablet; M-Cin, M-Floxin, Mois. 100 mg injection; M-Cin, Moxicip, Staxom.

PROTHINAMIDE

Dosage: PO—10–20 mg/kg/day once daily (maximum: 750 mg).

Brands: 250 mg tablet; Mycotuf-P, Prothicid.

Antispasmodics

chapter 22

These work by slowing the movements/spasms of the gut and other organs by relaxing the smooth muscles in the stomach and intestine; thus relieving the spasm and distension that causes pain. They may also cause constipation, dry mouth, drowsiness, and blurred vision.

DICYCLOMINE

Uses: Functional disturbances of gastrointestinal (GI) motility, renal colic.

Dosage: PO–infants >6 months: 5 mg/dose 3–4 times/day; children; 10 mg/dose 2 times/day (maximum: 20 mg/day). IM: 20 mg/dose.

Brands: 20 mg tablet; Coligon. 10 mg/mL injection; Centwin, Clomin.
Combinations:
- Dicyclomine 20 mg + PCM 500 mg tablet; Spasmoflexon, Spasmax
- Dicyclomine 10 mg + Dimethicone 40 mg: Per mL drop and per 5 mL suspension; Colimex
- Contraindicated in GI obstruction, tachycardia, urinary tract obstruction and infant <6 months of age. Children of Down syndrome, spastic paralysis or brain damage are more susceptible to adverse effects.

DROTAVERINE

Uses: As spasmolytic in nephrolithiasis, cholelithiasis, spastic constipation.

Dosage: 1–5 years: 20 mg 3 times/day; 6–12 years: 40 mg 3 times/day.

Brands: 40 and 30 mg tablet; Dotarin, Drotin, Drot. 20 mg/mL injection; Drot, Tavan 10 mg/5 mL suspension; Drotin.

HYOSCINE BUTYLBROMIDE

Uses: Spasmodic GI tract disorders, adjunctive therapy of peptic ulcer, hypermotility of lower urinary tract, infant colic.

Dosage: PO—children >6 years, 10–20 mg, 3 times/day injection; 5 mg 3 times/day.

Brands: 10 mg tablet; 20 mg/mL injection; 7.5 and 10 mg suppository; Buscopan.

- Contraindicated in megacolon, GI mechanical stenosis, tachycardia.

LACTASE ENZYME

Uses: Primary or secondary lactose intolerance related colic.

Dosage: PO
- 0–3 months: 20–30 drops/day in devided doses.
- >4 months: 4 drops/feed.

Breastfeed: Express 2–3 teaspoon of milk into a clean container. Add 2 drops of enzyme and then feed this to baby. Now continue breastfeed.

Formula feed: After preparing milk add 2 drops of enzyme, mix well then feed the baby. Discard the unused quantity.

Brands: 600 units/mL drops; Cry-No, Lactaze.

- Direct administration of lactase enzyme will be get destroyed by the gastric acid
- Do not exceed maximum dose per day.

PROPANTHELINE BROMIDE

Uses: Adjunctive therapy of pancreatitis, ureteral, and urinary bladder spasm, peptic ulcer.

Dosage: 1–2 mg/kg/day in 3–4 divided doses (maximum: 75 mg/day).

Brands: 15 mg tablet; Probanthine, Spastheline.

Antitoxins

chapter 23

An antibody that is produced in response to and are capable of neutralizing a specific biologic toxin, such as those that cause diphtheria, gas gangrene or tetanus are known as antitoxins. Antitoxins are used as both prophylactically and therapeutically. Antitoxins are produced by certain animals, plants, and bacteria in response to toxin exposure.

ANTISNAKE VENOM

Uses: Snakebite along with required medical management.

Dosage: IV
- Mild cases: 5 vials (50 mL).
- Moderate cases: 5–15 vials (50–150 mL).
- Severe cases: 15–20 vials (150–200 mL).
- Smaller children may require higher dose due to large dose of venom injected per unit bodyweight.

Brands: Available in lyophilized form and neutralizes Cobra, Russel's viper, Saw-scaled viper and krait venom. 10 mL Polyvalent injection; by BE, Bharat Serum, Haffkine.

Administration: If time permits, do exclude equine serum allergy by intradermal injection of 0.02 mL of 1:10 diluted antivenom. The antivenom is given diluted in 250 mL of normal saline at a rate of 20 mL/kg/h.
- Intramuscular adrenaline may be given before administering antisnake venom as prophylaxis.
- Anaphylaxis is to be treated with antihistamines, adrenaline. IV fluids, aminophylline, and oxygen.
- Immunization for tetanus is to be given in each and every case.

DIPHTHERIA ANTITOXIN/ANTIDIPHTHERIC SERUM

Uses: Diphtheria along with required medical management.

Dosage: Doses remain same in all age groups; IV–
- Nasal diphtheria: 20,000 IU
- Tonsillar and pharyngeal diphtheria: 40,000–80,000 IU
- Laryngeal diphtheria: 120,000 IU
- Severe disease of 3 days or more with neck swelling: 80,000–120,000 IU.

Brands: Enzyme refined globulin solution 10,000 IU/vial by Haffkine.

Administration: Test for hypersensitivity. Amount to be given is diluted in 1:20 isotonic normal saline (NS) and given at the rate of 1 mL/min.
- Diphtheria immunoglobulin (DIG) can be used in place of ADS in a dose of 0.6 mL/kg.
- Can be given IM in mild cases.

GAS GANGRENE ANTITOXIN

Uses: Gas gangrene infection caused by *Clostridium* bacteria.

Dosage: IV, IM, SC—30,000–75,000 IU.

Brands: 10,000 IU/vial; AGGS by Bharat Serum.

TETANUS ANTITOXIN

Uses: Prophylaxis and treatment of tetanus in cases where tetanus immunoglobulin is not available.

Dosage: IM, SC
- Prophylaxis <30 kg: 1,500 units. >30 kg: 3,000–5,000 units
- Treatment: 50,000–100,000 units.

Brands: 750, 1,500, 5,000, 10,000, 20,000, 50,000 IU injection by Bengal Immunity. 1,500, 10,000, 20,000, IU injection by Haffkine.

Administration: Should be given after sensitivity test. For treatment given half IV and half IM.

Antiulcers/ Antisecretory

chapter 24

PROTON PUMP INHIBITOR

These agents decrease gastric acid secretion by selectively inhibiting the proton pump, also demonstrate activity against *H. pylori*. These agents may cause constipation, headache, abdominal pain, dizziness, rash, leukopenia. Useful for duodenal ulcers, erosive gastritis, esophagitis, hypersecretory conditions, prevention and treatment of nonsteroidal anti-inflammatory drugs (NSAIDs) associated gastric ulcers, adjuvant therapy in the treatment of *H. pylori* infection. Administer before eating. Also available in combination with domperidone.

ESOMEPRAZOLE

Uses: Gastroesophageal reflux disease (GERD)
Dosage: PO—taken 1 hour before meal.
- Children <30 kg: 0.5–1 mg/kg once daily (maximum: 15 mg/day).
- Adolescents and children >30 kg: 20–40 mg once daily.

Brands: 20, 40 mg tablet; Esomac, Esotrax, Nexpro 15 mg sachet; Esole.

LANSOPRAZOLE

Dosage: PO—taken 1 hour before meal.
- Children <30 kg: 0.5–1 mg/kg (maximum 15 mg) once daily. 30 kg: 15–30 mg once daily.

Brands: 15 and 30 mg capsule; Lan, Lanzap, Lanzol.
- Decreases vitamin B_{12} absorption.

OMEPRAZOLE

Dosage: PO in >2 years of age: 0.6–0.7 mg/kg once daily. Titrate to desired effect.

Brands: 10 and 20 mg capsule; Lomac, Lomecid, Ocid.

PANTOPRAZOLE

Dosage: PO in >6 years of age: 0.5 mg/kg once daily.

Brands: 20 and 40 mg tablet; Lupipan, Pan, Pantocid.

SUCRALFATE

Uses: Duodenal and gastric ulcer, prevention of stress ulcer, NSAIDs associated mucosal damage, topically for chemotherapy-induced stomatitis, burns.

Dosage:
- PO—40–80 mg/kg/day divided q 6 hr. <2 years: 250 mg; 1–12 years: 500 mg; 12–18 years: 1 g 4–6 times/day.
- Stomatitis: 5–10 mL of 1 g/10 mL, Swish and spit or swish and swallow 4 times/day.

Brands: 0.5 g/5 mL; Sucral kid, Pepsigard-p. 1 g/5 mL syrup; Pepsigard, Sucral. 1 g tablet; Pepsigard, Sucral, Sucralfil.
- Interferes with absorption of vitamin A, D, E and K may cause constipation, dry mouth, hypophosphatemia, vertigo, headache.
- Use in preterm newborn, may lead to bezoar formation and subacute abstraction symptoms and should be avoided.

Antivirals

chapter 25

Most viral infections resolve spontaneously in immunocompetent individuals, aim of the therapy in viral infections is to minimize symptoms and infectivity, and shorten duration of illness. To maintain their growth and to reproduce, viruses must enter living cells. Thus, it is difficult to find a drug that is specific for the virus and that does not interfere with the function of host cell. Antivirals currently available acts by arresting the viral replication cycle at various stages of their growth. Unlike antimicrobials, antiviral does not deactivate or destroy the virus but act by inhibiting replication and thus decreasing viral load to non-pathogenic level.

ACYCLOVIR

Uses: Cutaneous herpes simplex, herpes simplex virus (HSV) encephalitis, herpes zoster vaccine (HZV) infection, varicella zoster.

Dosage:
- Neonatal herpes: 20 mg/kg/dose q 8 hr IV for 14–21 days
- HSV encephalitis: 10–20 mg/kg/dose q 8 hr IV for 14–21 days
- Genital herpes: PO—40–80 mg/kg/day divided q 8 hr for 5–7 days
- Recurrent or suppression of genital herpes: PO—40–80 mg/kg/day divided q 8 hr for 12 months
- Varicella zoster, initiate treatment within 24 hours of onset of rash: PO—20 mg/kg/dose, 4 times/day for 5 days.

Brands: 200, 400, 800 mg tablet; 25 mg/mL injection; Acivir, Axovir.
- Incompatible with blood products and protein containing solutions. Adequate hydration should be maintained during therapy. Administer slowly to prevent renal damage. Use with caution in liver disease and

epilepsy. Do not refrigerate solution because it can cause precipitation of the drug.

ADENINE

Uses: HSV infection.

Dosage: IV–neonatal HSV: 15–30 mg/kg/day once daily for 10–21 days. Infusion is given slowly over 12 hours.

Brands: 200 mg/vial, 3% eye ointment; Vira-A.

ADEFOVIR

Uses: Treatment of chronic hepatitis B

Dosage: PO—10 mg/day.

Brands: 10 mg tablet; Adesore, Adfovir.

AMANTADINE

Uses: Prophylaxis and treatment of influenza A virus infection.

Dosage: PO–5 mg/kg/day divided q 12 hr maximum 150 mg/day in 1–9 years and 200 mg/day in 10–20 years of age group.

Brands: 100 mg capsule; Amantrel, Neaman.

- Administer within 24–48 hour of onset of symptoms and duration of treatment is 2–5 days.

CIDOFOVIR

Uses: Cytomegalovirus (CMV) retinitis; CMV, HSV, VZV infections resistant to first-line drug; recurrent respiratory papillomatosis.

Dosage: IV:
- For CMV retinitis: 5 mg/kg/dose once by slow infusion
- Oral probenecid must be accompanied before and after IV cidofovir along with adequate normal saline (NS) hydration.

FAMCICLOVIR

Uses: HSV and VZV infection.

Dosage: PO—can be used in older children in a dose of 100 mg/kg three times/day (maximum: 200–500 mg/day) for 5–7 days.

Brands: 250 and 500 mg tablet; Famtrex, Penvir, Virovir.
- May cause urinary retention, hypotension, electrolyte imbalance.

FOSCARNET

Uses: Treatment of CMV, VZV infection resistant to first-line drug; CMV retinitis.

Dosage:
- CMV retinitis: Induction–180 mg/kg/day divided q 8 hr for 14–21 days. Maintenance—90–120 mg/kg/day once daily.
- Resistant HSV: 40 mg/kg/dose q 8 hr for 3 weeks.

Brands: 500 mg,1 g vial; Foscavir.

GANCICLOVIR

Uses: First choice drug for CMV infection, CMV retinitis, also active against HSV 1 and 2.

Dosage: Slow IV infusion–
- Congenital CMV infection: 15 mg/kg/day BD.
- CMV retinitis: >3 months–induction therapy; 10 mg/kg/ day twice a day for 14–21 days. Maintenance; 5 mg/kg/ day twice a day for 5 days in a week.
- Other CMV infection: Initial dose of 10–15 mg/kg/day twice a day for 14–21 days followed by 5 mg/kg/day single daily dose.
- Oral (following induction by IV): 30 mg/kg/dose q 8 hr with food.

Brands: 250 and 500 mg capsule; Ganguard, Ganvir 500 mg/vial; Cytogan, Gavir.
- Use with caution in patient with bone marrow suppression. May cause pancreatitis, hematuria, hypertension, electrolyte imbalance, neutropenia.

IDOXURIDINE

Uses: Topical therapy for herpes simplex keratitis.

Dosage: Apply ointment 5 times/day and solution 7–10 times/day.

Brands: 0.1% ointment; Toxil. 0.1% drop; Idurin, Ridinox.

INTERFERON ALFA

Uses and dosage: SC
- Hemangiomas of infancy: 1–3 million units/m^2/day once daily
- Chronic hepatitis B: 3–10 million units/m^2/day, 3 times/week
- Chronic hepatitis C: 3 million units/m^2/day, 3 times/week.

Brands: 3 million units/vial (alfa 2a); Intron-a, Roferon-A. 3 and 5 million units/vial (alfa 2b), Shanferon, Realfa.

- Use with caution in patient with seizure disorder, myelosuppression, asthma, renal impairment. Should not be used in autoimmune hepatitis.

ISOPRINOSINE

Uses: Subacute sclerosing panencephalitis.

Dosage: PO : 50-100 mg/kg/day in 2 divided doses.

Brand: 500 mg tablet; Isoprinosine.

LAMIVUDINE

Uses: HIV infection, chronic hepatitis B infection associated with evidence of viral replication and active liver inflammation.

Dosage: PO
- Neonates: 2 mg/kg/day divided q 12 hr
- Infants >3 months and children: 4 mg/kg/dose twice daily (maximum: 150 mg/dose)
- Chronic hepatitis B: 3 mg/kg/dose once daily (maximum: 100 mg/day).

Brands: 100 and 150 mg tablet; Lamivir, Lamuvid, Shanvudin.

- Use with caution in patients with pancreatitis, hepatic failure. May cause hypertension (HT), peripheral neuropathy, bone marrow suppression.

OSELTAMIVIR

Uses: Uncomplicated acute illness due to influenza A and B.

Dosage: Treatment should begin within 2 days of onset of symptoms.
PO—Children: 1–12 years: <15 kg, 30 mg BD; >15–23 kg, 45 mg bd; >23–40 kg: 60 mg bd; >40 kg: 75 mg bd; for 5 days.

Brands: 75 mg capsule;12 mg/mL suspension; Antiflu, Tamiflu.
- May cause anemia, hepatitis, myalgia, rash, hematuria.

RIBAVIRIN

Uses: RSV lower respiratory tract infection with compromising conditions, such as bronchopulmonary dysplasia (BPD), chronic lung disease (CLD), congenital heart disease (CHD); acute illness due to influenza A and B, adenovirus; oral preparation in combination with interferon alfa 2b in chronic hepatitis C in children >3 years of age.

Dosage: PO; inhalation–
- Aerosol inhalation (dissolve 6 g powder in 300 mL of sterile water). Continuous inhalation:12–18 hour/day for 3–7 days. Intermittent inhalation: 2 g over 2 hours, 3 times/day for 3–7 days.
- Oral: Chronic hepatitis C in children >3 years of age; 15 mg/kg/day divided q 12 hr (maximum: 200 mg BD).

Brands: 100 and 200 mg tablet; Virazide. 50 mg/5 mL syrup; Ribavin, Virazide.
- Do not use in patients of hemoglobinopathies, autoimmune hepatitis. Use in well-ventilated room, drug may precipitate in ventilator tubing, best results are seen in early initiation of treatment.

RIMANTADINE

Uses: Prophylaxis (all ages) and treatment (>13 years) of influenza A viral infection.

Dosage:
- Prophylaxis: 1–9 years up to 40 kg; 5 mg/kg/day divided q 12 hr (maximum: 150 mg/day). More than 10 years or above 40 kg; 100 mg in 2 divided dose.
- Treatment: 100 mg twice a day.

TRIFLURIDINE

Uses: Herpes simplex conjunctivitis and keratitis.

Dosage: Topical—1 drop in each eyes 8 times/day, following re-epitheliazation,1 drop 4 tmes/day. Total duration of therapy is 21 days.

Brands: 1% eye drop;Viroptic.

ZANAMIVIR

Uses: Treatment and prophylaxis of Infuenza.

Dosage: Inhalation–children >5 years: 10 mg twice daily for 5 days. Prophylaxis: 10 mg once daily for 7 days.

Brands: Inhaler, 5 mg/actuation; Relenza, Virenza.

Cardiac Shocks and Failures

chapter 26

AMRINONE

Uses: Treatment of low cardiac output states.

Dosage: Initial dose of 0.75 mg/kg over 2–3 minutes followed by 5–10 µg/kg/min as continuous infusion (maximum: 10 mg/kg/day).

Brands: 5 mg/mL injection; Amicor, Cardiotone.
- May cause hypotension, thrombocytopenia, dizziness, etc.
- Has vasodilatory and inotropic effect.

DIGOXIN

Uses: Treatment of systolic heart failure and supraventricular tachyarrhythmias.

Dosage: PO—Parenteral dose is 2/3 of this amount.
- Neonate: 10–30 µg/kg loading dose followed by 5–10 µg/kg/day as maintenance dose
- 1 month to 2 years: 30 µg/kg loading dose followed by 10–15 µg/kg/day as maintenance dose
- 2–10 years: 30 µg/kg loading dose followed by 5–10 µg/kg/day as maintenance dose
- >10 years: 10 µg/kg loading dose followed by 2–5 µg/kg/day as maintenance dose.
- Give half of the total digitalizing dose stat, then 1/4 after 8 hours and second 1/4 after 16 hours. Maintenance dose is given divided 12 hours in <10 years and once daily in >10 years of age. Nowadays, digitalization is not practiced routinely. Maximum PO dose is 250 µg; IV dose is 200 µg.

Brands: 0.25 mg tablet; Cardioxin, Digoxin, Dixin, Lanoxin. 0.25 mg/mL injection; Cardioxin, Digoxin, Dixin. 1.5 mg/mL syrup; Lanoxin.

Administration: Avoid rapid IV push, as it may cause systemic and coronary arteriolar vasoconstriction.

- May cause bradycardia, arrhythmias, blurred vision, gastrointestinal (GI) disturbances, vertigo, hypokalemia, diplopia
- Toxicity is enhanced by hypokalemia.
- Half life is markedly prolonged in preterm babies and in those with renal dysfunction.

MILRINONE

Uses: Short-term treatment of acute decompensated heart failure.

Dosage: IV—loading dose of 50 μg/kg given slowly over 15 minutes followed by a continuous infusion of 0.5 μg/kg/min.

Brands: 1 mg/mL injection; Milicor, Myolong.

- May cause arrhythmias, tremor, hypokalemia, rash.
- Has inotropic and vasodilatory action.

VASOPRESSIN

Uses: Diabetes insipidus, GI hemorrhage or esophageal varices bleed, vasodilatory shock with hypotension not responding to catecholamines or fluid resuscitation.

Dosages:
- Vasodilatory shock with hypotension: IV—0.0003–0.002 units/kg/minute titrate to effect
- Diabetes insipidus: IM, SC—2.5–10 units/dose can be given 2–4 times/day
- GI hemorrhage: Continuous IV infusion of 0.002–0.01 units/kg/min.

Brands: 20 units/mL injection; Petressin, Cpressin-P.

- Use with caution in patients of asthma, seizure disorder, cardiac disease. May cause hypertension, bradycardia, arrhythmias, vertigo, bronchoconstriction, sweating, tremor, water intoxication.
- For IV use dilute in D-5% or normal saline (NS) to a concentration of 0.2–1 unit/mL.

Chelating Agents

chapter 27

Chelating agents are chemical compounds that react with metal ions to form a stable, water soluble complex which are easily excreted.

DEFERIPRONE

Uses: Transfusional hemosiderosis, acute iron poisoning, iron overload in hemolytic anemia.

Dosage: PO—75 mg/kg/day divided q 8 hr

Brands: 250 and 500 mg tablet; Kelfer.
- May cause neutropenia, urine discoloration, musculoskeletal pain, gastrointestinal (GI) disturbances.

DEFERASIROX

Uses: Iron overload, thalassemia major, hemolytic anemia on multiple transfusion.

Dosage: PO—>2 years: Initially 20 mg/kg once daily empty stomach. Dose can be adjusted based on serum ferritin levels and can be increased every 3–6 months by 5–10 mg/kg (maximum: 30 mg/kg/day).

Brands: 250, 500 mg tablet; Desirox, Defrijet. 100, 200 mg tablet; Asunra, Desifer.

DESFERRIOXAMINE

Uses: Acute iron poisoning, chronic iron overload in patient requiring multiple blood transfusion, aluminiun overload.

Dosage:
- Acute iron intoxication: IM—90 mg/kg/dose q 8 hr. IV—15 mg/kg/hour (maximum: 6 g/day).
- Chronic iron overload: IV—15 mg/kg/h (maximum: 12 g/day). SC—20–40 mg/kg/day over 8–12 hours via infusion device. (maximum: 2g/day).

- In thalassemics: 15 mg/kg by IV infusion per unit of blood transfusion by separate line.
- Aluminium overload in dialysis patients: IV—infusion at 5 mg/kg once weekly via fistula over last 1 hour of hemodialysis or hemofiltration for 3 months.

Brands: 500 mg/vial; Desferal.

- May cause flushing, hypotension, urticaria, hearing loss, blurred vision, fever, urine discoloration. Periodic eye and auditory examinations are recommended while on chronic therapy.
- IV is given as 10% solution. Infusion rate must not exceed 15 mg/kg/hr to avoid hypotension.
- Therapy is continued till free iron is no longer present in the plasma or urinary screen for iron is negative.

DIMERCAPROL

Uses: Antidote to arsenic, gold, and mercury poisoning, adjunct in lead poisoning.

Dosage: Deep IM—2.5–4 mg/kg/dose q 4–6 hr for 2 days followed by 2.5 mg/kg dose q 12 hr for 10 days.

Brands: 100 mg/vial; BAL.

D-PENICILLAMINE

Uses: Wilson's disease, copper and lead poisoning, rheumatoid arthritis, cystinuria.

Dosage: PO
- Wilson's disease: 20 mg/kg/day in divided doses (maximum: 1g/day)
- Lead poisoning: 20–30 mg/kg/day in divided doses (maximum: 1.5 g/day); treatment duration 4–12 weeks
- Rheumatoid arthritis: 3 mg/kg/day for 3 months then 6 mg/kg/day in two divided doses for 3 months (maximum: 10 mg/kg/day).

Brands: 250 mg capsule; Cilamin, Distamin, Penamine.

- Pyridoxine in a dose of 25–50 mg/day should be supplemented while on D-penicillamine therapy.

Colony-stimulating Factors

chapter 28

Colony-stimulating factors are secreted glycoprotiens that bind to receptor on the surfaces of hemopoietic stem cells, thereby activating intracellular signaling pathways that can cause the cells to proliferate and differentiate into a specific kind of blood cells (usually white blood cells, but red blood cells in case of erythropoietin). The new blood cells formed migrate into the bloodstream and perform there function.

ERYTHROPOIETIN/rHuEPO/EPO

Uses: Anemia of prematurity, neoplasia, end-stage renal disease, chemotherapy induced, associated with AIDS and its therapy.

Dosage: IV, SC—dosing schedules need to be individualized.
- Anemia of prematurity: 100–500 units/kg/dose, 3 times/week
- Chronic renal failure: 50–100 units/kg/dose, 3 times/week
- Cancer patients: 150 units/kg/dose, 3 times/week
- Human immunodeficiency virus (HIV) patients: 100 units/kg/dose, 3 times/week.

Brands: 2,000 and 4,000 IU/vial; Epotin, Hemax.
- Iron, vitamin B_{12}, folic acid deficiency limits marrow response and EPO may be ineffective and these need to be supplemented. Avoid shaking the vial as this may denature the glycoprotein rendering it ineffective. May cause hypertension (HT), headache, seizure, edema, arthralgia.

FILGRASTIM

Uses: Prevention of febrile neutropenia and associated infection in patients who have received bone marrow and antineoplastics for the treatment of non-myeloid malignancies. Management of severe chronic neutropenia. Reduction of time for neutrophil recovery and duration of fever in patient undergoing induction and consolidation chemotherapy for acute myelogenous leukemia. Neonatal neutropenia.

Dosage: After myelosuppressive chemotherapy—children: IV/SC—5 µg/kg/day as a single SC injection for up to 2 weeks or until absolute neutrophil count (ANC) reaches 10,000/m^3. Initiate at least 24 hour after chemotherapy. Dose may be increased by 5 µg/day during each cycle of chemotherapy, depending on blood counts.
- Neonatal neutropenia: IV/SC—5–10 µg/kg/day once daily for 3–5 days.

Brands: 300 µg/vial; Cytograf, Grafeel.

GRANULOCYTE COLONY-STIMULATING FACTOR (G-CSF)

Uses: Neonatal, congenital and idiopathic neutropenia; patients with malignancies receiving drugs associated with severe neutropenia and fever.

Dosage: IV, SC
- Neonates: 5 µg/kg/day for 3–5 days once daily
- Children: 5–10 µg/kg/day once daily for up to 14 days.

Brands: 300 µg/mL vial; Neupogen.
- Do not administer 24 hour prior to or within 24 hours following chemotherapy. After discontinuation of therapy ANC decreases by 50% within 2 days and return to re-treatment level within 1 week, White blood count (WBC) count return to normal range in 4–7 days.

GRANULOCYTE-MACROPHAGE COLONY-STIMULATING FACTOR (GM-CSF)

Uses: Acceleration of myeloid recovery from chemotherapy or marrow insult or after bone marrow transplantation, neutropenia of preterm, neutropenia following ganciclovir therapy.

Dosage:
- Neonates: 10 µg/kg/day once daily for 5 days
- Children: 250 µg/m^2/day once daily for 21 days.

Brands: 500 µg/mL injection; Leukine.

PEGFILGRASTIM

Uses: To decrease the incidence of infection in patients with non-myeloid malignancies receiving myelosuppressive antineoplastics associated with a high-risk of febrile neytropenia.

Dosage: SC—children >45 kg: 6 mg/chemotherapy cycle.

Brands: 6 mg/vial; Neulastim, Peg-Grafeel.

Corticosteroids

chapter 29

Systemic steroids are contraindicated in active untreated infections and if required should be administered with food to decrease gastrointestinal gastrointestinal (GI) side effects. Taper gradually on long-term use. May cause edema, hypertension (HT), pseudotumor cerebri, Cushing's syndrome, pituitary-adrenal axis suppression, growth retardation, sodium retention, muscle weakness, osteoporosis, peptic ulcer. Topical use may cause thin fragile skin, hyper- or hypopigmentation, skin atrophy. Patient may require diet rich in potassium, calcium, zinc, vitamin A, B, C, D; low in sodium content. Do not apply occlusive dressing after topical use and do not apply to face or inguinal areas..Additional dose may be needed during stress. May mask signs of infection. Use lowest possible dose for shortest time possible. Alternate day therapy is preferable during long-term use.

BETAMETHASONE

Uses: Stimulate fetal lung maturation in preterm labor, congenital adrenal hyperplasia, brain edema, severe asthma; systemic and topical anti-inflammatory or immunosuppressant.

Dosage: Depends upon disease severity and patient response.
- IM, PO—0.01–0.2 mg/kg/day divided q 6–8 hr (maximum: 4 mg/day).
- Stimulate lung maturation: IM, given to pregnant mother in 2 doses of 12 mg q 24 hr or four doses of 6 mg q 12 hr
- Topical: Apply thin film 1–2 times/day.

Brands: 0.5 and 1 mg tablet; Betnesol, Cortil. 0.5 mg/mL oral drops; 4 mg/mL injection; Betnesol, Celestone, Stemin. 0.05% cream; Betamil, Diprovate.

CLOBETASONE

Uses: Atopic dermatitis, corticosteroid responsive dermatoses.

Dosage: Topically apply a thin film 2–3 times daily on affected area for a maximum period of 2 weeks.

Brands: 0.05% cream; Eumosone, Fembesol, Sterisone.

CORTISONE

Uses: Adrenocortical insufficiency.

Dosage: PO—0.5–0.7 mg/kg/day divided q 8 hr; IM—0.25–0.35 mg/kg/day.

Brands: 25 mg tablet; 50 mg/mL injection; Cortone. 5,25 mg tablet; Cortin. 25 mg tablet; Cortisyl.

DEFLAZACORT

Uses: Juvenile chronic arthritis (polyarticular disease), asthma, nephrotic syndrome, immunosuppression in transplantation.

Dosage: PO– usual range is 0.25–1.5 mg/kg/day in divided doses.
- 1 month to 12 years: 250 µg to 1.5 mg/day in divided doses.
- 12–18 years: 2–18 mg/day in divided doses.

Brands: 1, 6, 24 mg tablet; Defcort, Defnalon, Dezacort, Enzocort.
- Use the lowest effective doses and titrate dose depending upon response. Alternate day administration may be appropriate.
- Antacids should not be given 2 hours prior or after administration of deflazacort. Deflazacort 6 mg is equivalent to 5 mg of prednisolone.

DEXAMETHASONE

Uses: Cerebral edema, septic shock, bacterial meningitis; systemically and locally for inflammation; allergic, autoimmune and neoplastic diseases.

Dosage:
- Physiologic replacement: PO, IM, IV—0.03–0.15 mg/kg/ day divided q 6–12 hr
- Cerebral edema: PO, IM, IV—loading dose of 1–2 mg/kg, then 1–1.5 mg/kg/day divided q 4–6 hr

- Bacterial meningitis: IV—0.6 mg/kg/day divided q6h for first 4 days of antibiotic
- Anti-inflammatory: PO, IM, IV—0.05–0.5 mg/kg/day in divided doses
- Congenital adrenal hyperplasia (CAH) after completion of linear growth: PO—0.5–1 mg/day.
- Acute attack of asthma: IM—0.6 mg/kg single dose daily for 2 days.
- Topical: Apply thin film 1–2 times/day
- Eye drop: 1–2 drop q 4 hr then taper off gradually.

Brands: 0.5 mg tablet; 4 mg/mL injection; Decdan, Dexacip, Dexona, Wymosone. 0.5, 0.75, 1, 1.5, 2, 4, 6 mg tablet; Decadron, Decdon, Dexarone. 0.1% cream; Millicortenol. 0.01% eye drop; Decolite, Losone.

FLUDROCORTISONE

Use: Partial replacement therapy for adrenal insufficiency.

Dosage: 0.05–0.1 mg/day single oral dose.

Brands: 100 µg tablet; Floricot, Florinef.

HYDROCORTISONE

Uses: Adrenal insufficiency, congenital adrenal hyperplasia, toxic shock, status asthmaticus, anti-inflammatory or immunosuppressive in dermatosis.

Dosage: IV
- Adrenal insufficiency: 1–2 mg/kg bolus followed by 25–150 mg/day in divided doses
- Congenital adrenal hyperplasia: Initial dose of 0.5–0.7 mg/day followed by maintenance dose of 0.3–0.4 mg/ kg/day; given ¼ in morning, ¼ at noon and ½ at night
- Shock: Initial dose of 35–50 mg/kg followed by 50–150 mg/kg/day divided q 6 hr for 2–3 days
- Status asthmaticus: 4–8 mg/kg/day in divided doses
- Anti-inflammatory: 1–5 mg/kg/day divided q 12 hr
- Topical: Apply 2–3 times/day.

Brands: 100 mg/vial; Efcorlin, Hycort, Lycortin, Wycort. 0.1% cream; Elderoid, Lipo. 0.5% cream; Tendrone. 2.5% ointment; Wycort.

METHYLPREDNISOLONE

Uses: Anti-inflammatory or immunosuppressant in variety of allergic, inflammatory, autoimmune and neoplastic disorders; acute spinal cord injury, idopathic thrombocytopenic purpura (ITP).

Dosage:
- Anti-inflammatory or immunosuppressant: PO, IM, IV—0.5–2 mg/kg/day in divided doses. Pulse therapy:15–30 mg/kg/dose given slowly once daily for 3 days.
- Status asthmaticus: IV—loading dose of 2 mg/kg/dose then 0.5–1 mg/kg/dose q 6 hr.
- Acute spinal cord injury: IV—30 mg/kg over 15 minutes followed 45 minutes later by continuous infusion of 5 mg/kg/h for 1 day.
- Shock: IV—30 mg/kg/dose every 6 hours for 2–3 days.

Brands: 4, 8, and 16 mg tablet; Ivepred, Medrol, Predmet. 40, 125, 500 mg and 1 g injection; Mypred, Solu-medrol, Succimed.

MOMETASONE

Uses: As anti-inflammatory and antipruritic in eczema, atopic and contact dermatitis; psoriasis; allergic rhinitis, nasal polyps, obstructive sleep apnea in children >2 years of age.

Dosage: Allergic rhinitis, nasal polyps, obstructive sleep apnea–one spray of 50 µg/dose into each nostril once daily in >2 years of age and in >12 years of age it is two sprays into each nostril once a day.
- Cream and ointment >2 years: Apply a thin film to affected area BD. Safety and efficacy for >3 weeks use is not established in pediatric patients.

Brands: 50 µg/sparay; Furomet, Momeflo, Momate. 0.1% cream and ointment; Cutizone, Elocon, Momtas.
- Avoid contact/application to face, eyes, underarms, groin, and open skin.

PREDNISOLONE

Uses: Treatment of rheumatic carditis, infantile spasms, collagen diseases, skin diseases, allergic problem, nephrotic syndrome, asthma, endocrine and neoplastic disorders.

Dosage: Depends upon disease severity and patient response:
- Use alternate day therapy for prolonged use
- PO; IV—0.5–2 mg/kg/day divided q 6–8 hr.

Brands: 5, 10, and 20 mg tablet; Predone, Prid, Wysolone. 5 mg/5 mL syrup; Kidpred, Predone. 40 mg/mL injection; Unidrol, MPA.

TRIAMCINOLONE

Uses: Various allergic and inflammatory conditions.

Dosage:
- 6–12 years: IM—0.03–0.2 mg/kg q 1–7 days. Intra-articular, intrabursal; 2.5–15 mg may be repeated as needed.
- >12 years of age: PO—4–50 mg/day in divided doses.

Brands: 4 mg tablet; Kenacort, Ledercort, Tricort. 10 and 40 mg/mL injection; Comcort, Kenacort, Tricort.

Diuretics

chapter 30

Diuretics sometimes also called as water pills, are medications designed to increase the amount of water and salt expelled from the body as urine. There are mainly three types of diuretics, i.e., loop acting diuretics (Bumetanide), potassium sparing diuretics (Amiloride) and thiazide diuretics (Chlorothiazide). Other diuretics which does not fall into these groups, e.g., mannitol, etc. These are used for treatment of high BP, edema, heart and liver failure, etc.

ACETAZOLAMIDE

Uses: Diuretic, reduce cerebrospinal fluid (CSF) production in hydrocephalus, reduce increased intraocular pressure in glaucoma, as adjunct in refractory seizures, high altitude sickness.

Dosage: PO
- Edema: 5 mg/kg/day once daily
- Refractory seizures and glaucoma: 8–30 mg/kg/day in divided doses
- Hydrocephalus: 25–75 mg/kg/day divided q 8 hr.

Brands: 250 mg tablet; Acetamide, Diamox.
- Furosemide is used along with acetazolamide in hydrocephalus. May cause drowsiness, hypokalemia, hyperchloremic metabolic acidosis, hyperglycemia, dysuria, hepatic insufficiency.

AMILORIDE

Uses: Edema due to congestive heart failure (CHF), hepatic cirrhosis and hyperaldosteronism, hypertension.

Dosage: PO—6–20 kg– 0.6 mg/kg/day once daily (maximum: 10 mg/day). >20 kg: 5–10 mg/day (maximum: 20 mg/day).

Brands: Amiloride 2.5 mg + Hydrochlorothiazide 25 mg; Biduret tablets.

Combinations: Amiloride + Hydrochlorothiazide: 5 + 50 mg, 2.5 + 25 mg tablet; Biduret and Biduret-L.

- May cause hypotension, palpitation, headache, electrolyte imbalances, dehydration, muscle cramps, visual disturbances.

BUMETANIDE

Uses: Edema or fluid overload secondary to CHF, renal or hepatic disease.

Dosage: PO—0.015–0.1 mg/kg/dose q 6–24 hr (maximum: 10 mg/day).

Brands: 1 mg tablet, Bumet, Bumex, Burinex.

- May cause electrolyte imbalances, hyperglycemia, hypotension, dizziness, gastrointestinal (GI) disturbances. 1 mg of bumetanide is as potent as 40 mg of furosemide.

CHLORTHALIDONE

Uses: Fluid overload and mild hypertension.

Dosage: PO—1–2 mg/kg once daily.

Brands: 100 mg tablet; Hythalton. 12.5 mg tablet; Thalidone.

ETHACRYNIC ACID

Uses: Edema due to renal or hepatic disease, CHF, and hypertension.

Dosage: PO—1–3 mg/kg/day; IV—0.5–1 mg/kg/dose q 8–24 hr.

Brands: 50 mg tablet; 50 mg/vial; Edecrin.

- May cause hypotension, headache, fluid and electrolyte imbalances, ototoxicity, tinnitus.

FUROSEMIDE

Uses: Edema associated with CHF and hepatic or renal disease; hypertension, cerebral edema, forced diuresis in poisoning.

Dosage:
- IV—1–2 mg/kg/dose q 6–12 hr
- PO—1–4 mg/kg/dose q 6–12 hr
- Continuous infusion: 0.05 mg/kg/h and titrate to response.

Brands: 40 mg tablet; 10 mg/mL injection; Frusenex, Lasix.
- May cause hypotension, dizziness, fluid, and electrolyte imbalance, ischemic hepatitis.

HYDROCHLOROTHIAZIDE

Uses: Mild to moderate hypertension, edema states due to CHF, bronchopulmonary dysplasia, prevention of recurrent renal calcium stones.

Dosage:
- Neonates and infants <6 months: 2–4 mg/kg/day divided q 12 hr
- Infants >6 months and children: 2 mg/kg/day divided q 12 hr.

Brands: 12.5 and 25 mg tablet; Aquazide, Hydride.

MANNITOL

Uses: Reduction of increased intracranial pressure (ICP), promotion of diuresis in the prevention and treatment of oliguria or anuria due to acute renal failure (ARF), hyponatremia and water intoxication, peripheral edema, and ascites.

Dosage: IV—test dose of 200 mg/kg (over 3–5 minutes to evaluate urine output of at least 1 mL/kg/h for 1–3 hours) followed by initial dose of 0.5–1 g/kg, then maintenance dose of 0.25–0.5 g/kg q 4–6 hours.
- Cerebral and ocular edema: IV—initially 0.5–1 g/kg over 30 minutes followed by maintenance dose of 0.25–0.5 g/kg every 4–6 hours as required.
- Peripheral edema and ascites: IV infusion of 1–2 g/kg over 2–4 hours.

Brands: 20% mannitol is available in 100 mL bottles by Albert David, Cadila and Core.
- Contraindicated in severe renal disease, dehydration, active intracranial bleed, severe pulmonary edema or congestion.

METOLAZONE

Uses: Resistant cases of HT and heart failure.

Dosage: PO—0.2–0.4 mg/kg/day

Brands: 2.5, 5, 10 mg tablet; Diurem, Metiz, Zyntanix.
- Electrolytes must be monitored closely. Intermittent doses of metolazone may help to overcome diuretic resistance which may occur due to fluid overload and low renal blood flow.

SPIRONOLACTONE

Uses: Hypertension, edema associated with CHF, chronic liver disease, and nephrotic syndrome.

Dosage: PO—1–3 mg/kg/day once daily or in divided doses.

Brands: 25 and 100 mg tablet; Aldactone.
- May cause fluid and electrolyte imbalances, GI disturbance, numbness or paresthesia of limbs.

TORSEMIDE

Uses: Cardiac failure, pulmonary edema, HT, renal failure, fluid overload due to other causes.

Dosage:
- PO/IV—edema: 10–20 mg once daily (maximum: 200 mg/dose).
- HT—5–10 mg once daily.

Brands: 10, 20, 100 mg tablet; Divrator, Dytor, Metor. 10 mg/mL injection; Dytor.

TRIAMTERENE

Uses: Hypertension, edema due to CHF, hepatic or renal disease.

Dosage: PO—2–4 mg/kg/day divided q 12 hr (maximum: 6 mg/kg/day).

Brands:
- Triamterene 50 mg + Benzthiazide 25 mg: Ditide tablet
- Triamterene 50 mg + Furosemide 40 mg: Frusemene tablet.

Drugs Used for Controlling Bleeding

chapter 31

AMINOCAPROIC ACID

Uses: Treatment of excessive bleeding resulting from systemic hyperfibrinolysis or urinary fibrinolysis, traumatic ocular hyphema.

Dosage: PO, IV–loading dose of 100–200 mg/kg, maintenance dose is 100 mg/kg q 6 hr (maximum 30 g). In traumatic hyphema: 100 mg/kg q 4 hr.

Brands: 500 mg tablet; 250 mg/mL injection; Hemostat.
- Contraindicated in disseminated intravascular coagulation (DIC). May cause hypotension, bradycardia, headache, seizure, hypokalemia, nasal congestion.

ANTIHEMOPHILIC FACTOR

Uses: Factor VIII deficiency in hemophilia A.

Dosage: IV—20–50 U/kg/dose q 12 hr and titrate to required effect.

Brands: 25 IU vial; Factor VIII.

ETHAMSYLATE

Uses: Prevention and treatment of periventricular hemorrhage in low birth weight (LBW) neonates.

Dosage: Neonates; IM, IV–12.5 mg/kg q 6 hr.

Brands: 250 and 500 mg tablet; 125 mg/mL injection; Dicynene, Ethasyl, Sylate.
- Not helpful in thrombocytopenia.

FACTOR IX

Uses: Factor IX deficiency, hemophilia B, factor VIII inhibitors.

Dosage: IV—20–25 units/kg/dose once daily.
- In factor VIII inhibitor patients 75–100 units/kg/dose.

PROTAMINE

Uses: Antidote to bleeding due to heparin overdose.

Dosage: 1 mg of protamine neutralizes 100 units of heparin (low molecular weight heparin) (maximum: 50 mg). Adjust the protamine dosage depending upon the duration of heparin administration.

Time since last heparin dose	Dose of protamine to neutralize 100 units of heparin
<30 minutes	1 mg
30–60 minutes	0.5–0.75 mg
60–120 minutes	0.3–0.5 mg

Brands: 1% injection; Protamine sulfate.
- Excess dosage should be avoided as it can itself cause anticoagulation.

TRANEXAMIC ACID

Uses: Prevention of excessive bleeding after tonsillectomy, dental excretion, recurrent epistaxis, short-term use in hemophilia, prevention of GI hemorrhage and hemorrhage following ocular trauma, von Willebrand disease, thrombolytic overdose.

Dosage: IV—10 mg/kg/dose. PO—25 mg/kg/dose 3–4 times/day.

Brands: 500 mg tablet; 100 mg/mL injection; Clip, Pause, Tranfib, Traxamic.
- For IV use dilute with 5% dextrose or normal saline (NS). Can be mixed with heparin.

Supplements and Fluid Replacements

chapter 32

CALCIUM GLUCONATE

Uses: *Hypocalcemia, hyperkalemia*, cardiac arrest in the presence of *hyperkalemia or hypocalcemia* or calcium channel blocking agents toxicity.

Dosage: IV, 10% solution (100 mg/mL) is equivalent to 9 mg elemental calcium/mL or 0.46 mEq calcium/mL.
- Hypocalcemia: 200–800 mg/kg/day as continuous infusion or in four divided doses
- Cardiac arrest and hyperkalemia: 60–100 mg/kg/dose. (maximum: 3 g/dose).

Brands: 10% solution for injection; Calcium gluconate.
- IV solution should be diluted to 50 mg/mL and be given slowly over 1 hour under monitoring. Use with caution in patient on digitalis therapy. May cause hypotension, bradycardia, arrhythmias, hypercalcemia, hypophosphatemia.

CALCIUM PHOSPHATE

Uses: Calcium deficiency states, rickets, chronic renal failure.

Dosage: PO
- Neonate: 20–80 mg/kg/day divided doses
- Children: 45–65 mg/kg/day divided doses.

Brands: Ostocalcium syrup each 5 mL contains calcium 82 mg + Vitamin D_3 200 units + Vitamin B_{12} 2.5 µg. Ostocalcium tablet contains 125 mg of elemental calcium + Vitamin D_3 400 unit. Sovical L syrup each 5 mL contain elemental calcium 200 mg + Vitamin D_3 200 U.

MAGNESIUM SULFATE

Uses: Treatment of hypomagnesemia, hypertension, seizures associated with acute nephritis in children, adjunctive therapy in bronchodilatation.

Dosage: IV; 50% solution (500 mg/mL) is equivalent to 49 mg elemental magnesium/mL or 4 mEq/mL.

- Hypomagnesemia: 25–50 mg/kg/dose q 8 hr in neonates and q 6 hr in children for 3–4 doses (maximum: 2,000 mg)
- Seizures and hypertension: 20–100 mg/kg/dose q 4–6 hr as required
- Bronchodilator: 25 mg/kg/dose as single dose (maximum: 2,000 mg).

Brands: 50% solution for injection; Magnesium sulfate.

- Dilute to 50–200 mg/mL for IV use and infuse over 2–4 hours. Use with caution in digitalized and renal impairment patient. May cause hypotension, hypermagnesemia, gastrointestinal (GI) disturbances, central nervous system (CNS) depression, muscle weakness, respiratory paralysis.

POTASSIUM CHLORIDE

Uses: Hypokalemia; prevention and treatment.

Dosage: IV doses should be added to maintenance fluids and PO doses should be diluted to eight times in water.

- Hypokalemia: PO, IV—2–5 mEq/kg/day in divided doses
- Prevention of hypokalemia during diuretic therapy: PO—1–2 mEq/kg/day in two divided doses.

Brands: 600 mg tablet; Kgard. 10% syrup; Keylyte, Potasol. 15% ampule for injection; Potassium chloride.

- Rapid administration may cause arrhythmias and cardiac arrest, hypotension. Injectable should only be given in patient with adequate urine flow. Tablet provide 8 mEq; injection; 2 mEq/mL and syrup; 20 mEq/15 mL (1.5 g KCL).

DEXTROSE

Uses: To correct hypoglycemia, provide calories and fluid replacement, as adjunctive in treatment of hyperkalemia.

Dosage: IV

- Hyperkalemia: 0.5–1 g/kg of 25% or 50% solution combined with 1 unit of regular insulin for every 5 g dextrose, to be infused over 2 hours

- Hypoglycemia: Neonates; 0.1–0.2 g/kg/dose (1–2 mL/kg/dose of 10% solution) followed by 4–6 mg/kg/min. Infants and children: 0.5–1 g/kg/dose (2–4 mL/kg/dose of 25% solution).

SODIUM BICARBONATE

Uses: Metabolic acidosis, life-threatening hyperkalemia, correction of acid-base imbalance in cardiac arrest.

Dosage: 7.5% solution (75 mg/mL) is equivalent to 0.9 mEq/ mL. If acid-base status is not available then in older children empirical dose is 1–2 mEq/kg of 7.5% solution. Subsequent dose is calculated as follows:
- HCO_3 (mEq) = Base deficit × Weight in kilogram × 0.6
- Patient should be adequately ventilated before administering sodium bicarbonate in cardiac arrest.

Brands: 7.5% ampule for injection; Sodium bicarbonate.
- Contraindicated in hypocalcemia, hypernatremia, inadequate ventilation. May cause cerebral hemorrhage, metabolic alkalosis, hypernatremia, hypokalemia, hypocalcemia, pulmonary edema. For IV use dilute in equal volume of sterile water.

SODIUM CHLORIDE

Uses: Hyponatremia, restores moisture to nasal membrane, cystic fibrosis.

Dosage: Normal saline (0.9%) is equivalent to 154 mEq/L and 3% NaCl is equivalent to 513 mEq/L.
- Acute symptomatic hyponatremia: Given as follows–sodium (mEq) = Weight in kilogram × 0.6 × (desired sodium—actual sodium).
- In asymptomatic cases correct gradually as compared to symptomatic ones. Hypertonic NaCl should only be used for acute symptomatic hyponatremia. Dosage may vary depending upon fluid, electrolyte and acid-base balance coupled with clinical conditions.

Brands: 0.9 and 3% injection; NaCl. 0.9% nasal spray; 0.65% gel for nasal application; Nasoclear.
- Hypertonic saline should be given via central line only. For acute correction use 125 mEq/L as the desired sodium level.

H$_2$ Antagonists

chapter 33

These drugs inhibits the action of histamine at H$_2$-receptor site located primarily at gastric parietal cells, resulting in inhibition of gastric acid secretion.

CIMETIDINE

Uses: Treatment and prophylaxis of duodenal and gastric ulcers, gastroesophageal reflux, to prevent gastrointestinal (GI) hemorrhage in critically ill patients, hypersecretory conditions (Zollinger–Ellison syndrome).

Dosage: PO—infants and children—10–30 mg/kg/day divided q 6–12 hr.

Brands: 200 and 400 mg tablet; Cimetiget, Tymidin, Ulciban.

FAMOTIDINE

Uses: Same as cimetidine.

Dosage: PO, IV—0.5–1 mg/kg/day at bedtime or in two divided doses (maximum: 40 mg/day).

Brands: 20 and 40 mg tablet; 20 mg/mL injection; Famocid, Famonite.
- May cause palpitations, dizziness, thrombocytopenia, cholestatic jaundice.
- IV dose should be diluted to 4 mg/mL.

RANITIDINE

Uses: Same as cimetidine.

Dosage:
- Neonates: PO, IV—1.5–2 mg/kg/day q 12 hr
- Children: PO, IV; IM—1–5 mg/kg/day q 6–8 hr (maximum: 150 mg).

Brands: 150 and 300 mg tablet; 25 mg/mL injection; Aciloc, Histac, Ranitin, Rantac, Zinetac.

Immunoglobulins

chapter 34

HUMAN ANTI-D (Rho-D) IMMUNOGLOBULIN

Uses:
- Suppression of Rh isoimmunization (in mother): Used when the mother is Rho (D)-negative, father is either Rho (D)-positive or Rho (D) unknown, baby is either Rho (D)-positive or Rho (D) unknown. During delivery of Rho (D)-positive infant, abortion, chorionic villus sampling, amniocentesis, abdominal trauma, ruptured tubal pregnancy, transplacental hemorrhage.
- Treatment of idiopathic thrombocytopenic purpura (ITP): Used in Rho (D)-positive non-splenectomized children with acute or chronic ITP (investigational).

Dosage: IM–
- Pregnancy: 300 µg at 28 weeks and following delivery, preferably within 72 hours of delivery
- Postpartum: 300 µg within 72 hours
- Threatened abortion: 300 µg as soon as possible
- Abortion, miscarriage, termination of ectopic pregnancy. <13 weeks: 100 µg and ≥13 weeks: 300 µg within 72 hours.

Brands: 300 µg/vial; Gyne-D, Rhesuman, Rhogam.
- It has no role in already sensitized Rho (D)-negative women. Use with precautions in patient with bleeding disorders or thrombocytopenia or patient with hemoglobin <8 g%.

HUMAN CYTOMEGALOVIRUS (CMV) IMMUNOGLOBULIN

Uses: Acute CMV infection, CMV prophylaxis following transplant, AIDS, etc.

Dosage: IV–prophylaxis: 200 mg/kg pre-transplant; 100 mg/kg on days 7, 21, 42 and 63.
- Treatment: 200 mg/kg on days 1 and 7 given with appropriate antiviral therapy.
- Reconstitute a vial in 60 mL of distilled water provided with the pack. Contraindicated in selective IgA deficiency patients who posses antibody to IgA.

HUMAN HEPATITIS B IMMUNOGLOBULIN

Uses: Prophylaxis of hepatitis B in babies born to HBsAg-positive mothers, children acutely exposed to HBsAg-positive blood or blood products.

Dosage: IM
- Neonates: First dose of 100–200 IU given soon after delivery, followed by second dose of 32–48 IU/kg after 2–3 months. Hepatitis B vaccine should be given concurrently
- Children: 32–48 IU/kg soon after exposure.

Brands: 100 IU/0.5 mL; Hepabig, Hepaglob.

HUMAN NORMAL IMMUNOGLOBULIN (IVIG)

Uses: Immunodeficiency syndrome, ITP, Kawasaki disease, Guillain-Barre syndrome, acute bacterial or viral infections in immunosuppressed patient, demyelinating neuropathy, pediatric HIV infection, myocarditis, intractable epilepsy (myoclonus, tonic and atonic not resonding to drugs).

Dosage: IM, IV
- Immunodeficiency: 300–400 mg/kg/dose q 2–4 weeks; maintain IgG level >500 mg/dL.
- ITP: 400–1,000 mg/kg/day for 2–5 days then q 3–6 weeks based on platelet count and clinical response.
- Kawasaki disease: 2 g/kg single dose over 8–12 hours period. Treatment should be given within 7 days of onset of illness.
- Guillain-Barre syndrome: 400 mg/kg/day for 4 days.
- Myocarditis: 2 g/kg, given over 2 days.

- Intactable epilepsy: 400 mg/kg once in 3 weeks for 3 doses. If 75% reduction achieved, continue therapy for 9-12 months and review.
- Severe systemic viral or bacterial infection:
  - Neonates: 500 mg/kg/day for 2 days
  - Children: 500–1,000 mg/kg/week.

Brands: 0.5, 1, 2.5 and 5 g/vial; Gamma IV, Intraglobin CP, IV-Globulin.

- Doses should be based on ideal body weight. Protection usually lasts for 1–3 months.
- Contraindicated in patients with selective IgA deficiency who posses antibody to IgA.

HUMAN RABIES IMMUNOGLOBULIN (HRIG)

Uses: All proven and suspected rabid animal bite/exposure.

Dosage: IM and infilteration: 20 units/kg (maximum: 3,000 IU).

Brands: 300 IU/vial; Berirab-P, Imogam rabies, Rabglob. 750 IU/vial; Berirab-P.

Administration: If patient reports within 24 hour of exposure, give maximum dose for infiltration and rest is given IM over deltoid. If reports after 24 hours to 7 days then give total dose IM. Do skin sensitivity test. Rabies vaccine should be used concurrently.

HUMAN TETANUS IMMUNOGLOBULIN

Uses: Prophylaxis in non-immunized children and treatment of tetanus.

Dosage:
- Prophylaxis: 250 IU; IM or 4 units/kg. 500 IU, IM in case 24 hours have elapsed, wound is heavily contaminated and following burns.
- Treatment: 3,000–6,000 IU; IM and/or 250 IU intrathecal.

Brands: 250 and 500 IU injection: Immunotant, Tetglob.

RESPIRATORY SYNCYTIAL VIRUS IMMUNOGLOBULIN INTRAVENOUS (RSV-IGIV)

Uses: Prophylaxis in infants and children with severe immunodeficiency or immunosuppression; RSV infection in children <2 years of age with bronchopulmonary dysplasia or history of prematurity.

Dosage: IV—750 mg/kg given monthly from the beginning to the end of RSV infection season.

Brands: 50 mg/mL injection; Respigam.
- Immunization with live viral vaccine should be avoided for 9 months.

VARICELLA ZOSTER IMMUNOGLOBULIN (VZIG)

Uses: Prophylaxis in immunocompromised children, newborn exposed to maternal varicella, pregnant women.

Dosage: IM—125 units/kg soon after exposure or within 96 hours (maximum: 625 units).

Brands: >25 IU/mL injection; Varitect CP. 125 units/vial; VZIG.

Laxatives/Stool Softeners

chapter 35

Stool softener agents are used for acute or chronic constipation or to evacuate bowel before surgery, radiologic or endoscopic procedures. Contraindicated in persistent abdominal pain, nausea or vomiting of unknown cause, especially if accompanied by fever or other signs of an acute abdomen. Excessive or prolonged use may lead to dependence.

BISACODYL

Uses: Constipation, bowel cleansing.

Dosage:
- PO: 3–12 years: 5–10 mg single dose/day and >12 years: 5–15 mg single dose/day
- Rectal: <2 years, 5 mg/day and >2 years, 5–10 mg/day single dose.
- Preperation for surgery or radiological procedure: PO—<10 years, 5 mg; >10 years, 5–10 mg at bedtime for 2 days prior to procedure and rectally, if necessary, 1 hour before procedure.

Brands: 5 mg tablet; Dulcolax, Julax, Relax. 5 and 10 mg rectal suppository; Dulcolax, Conlax.
- Do not use in patient with abdominal pain, obstruction, appendicitis. Should not be used regularly for more than a week.
- Tablet acts in 10–12 hours, suppositories produce a motion within 20 minutes to 1 hour of insertion.

DOCUSATE

Uses: Habitual and opioid induced constipation, abdominal surgery.

Dosage: PO—in >6 months is recommended. <6 years: 20–40 mg/day and in >6 years 20–60 mg/day in 1–4 doses. Rectal: 3 to 18 years; 50 to 100 mg added to a retention or flushing enema once a day.

Brands: 100 mg tablet; 50 mg/5 mL syrup; 0.25% solution in 50 mL pack; Laxicon, Cellubril.
- Should not be used along with liquid paraffin.
- Rectally acts within 20 minutes.

ISPAGHULA HUSK

Uses: Constipation, Irritable bowel syndrome, spastic colon, ulcerative colitis.

Dosage: PO—child 2–12 years—1 level 5 mL spoonful in water once or twice daily. Child 12–18 years—2 level 5 mL spoonful in water once or twice daily, preferably at meal times.

Brands: 66 g husk/100 g; Igol, Feel good, Flow best.

LACTULOSE

Uses: Constipation, hepatic encephalopathy and coma.

Dosage: PO–infants—2.5–10 mL/day and in children 40–90 mL/day in 3–4 divided doses. Hepatic encephalopathy: Initially, 30–50 mL/dose 3 times/day. Then adjust dose to produce 2–3 soft stools/day.

Brands: 10 g/15 mL liquid; Duphalac, Evict, Lactulax.
- Target in hepatic encephalopathy is to produce 2–3 soft stools/day. Contraindicated in galactosemia or patient requiring low galactose diet. There occurs accumulation of hydrogen gas in intestine during therapy, could result in explosion if patient were to undergo electrocautery procedure.

LIQUID PARAFFIN

Uses: Constipation.

Dosage: PO—in children >18 months; initial 1 mL/kg can be increased up to 3 mL/kg once daily.

Brands: Liquid paraffin + Milk of magnesia—3.75 mL + 11.25 mL per 15 mL; Cremaffin, Cremalax, Trulax.
- Chronic use leads to deficiency of fat-soluble vitamins.
- Do not use when abdominal pain, nausea or vomiting are present.

POLYETHYLENE GLYCOL

Uses: Functional constipation.

Doses: PO—0.75–1.5 g/kg mixed in 200 mL of water or juice, can be given upto 2 weeks. It may take 2–4 days for the drug to produce a bowel movement.

Brands: 17 g sachet; 225 g jar; 3.35 g suspension; Laxopeg. 118 g sachet; Peglec.

SODIUM PICOSULFATE

Uses: Constipation, bowel cleansing before surgery or radiological procedures, opiod-induced constipation.

Dosage: PO–given at bedtime diluted with water. 2–5 years: 2.5 mL; 5–9 years: 2.5–5 mL; >10 years: 5–15 mL.

Brands: 10 mg tablet—Cremalax 5 mg/5 mL syrup; Laxcil, Laxobin.

- Contraindicated in undiagnosed abdominal pain or when intestinal obstruction is suspected.

Minerals

chapter 36

Minerals are solid substances that are present in nature and can be made of one element or more elements combined together. Minerals are naturally occurring. We will be discussing essential minerals.

FLUORIDE

Uses: Prevention of dental caries.

Dosage: Toothpaste once a day, rinse once or twice weekly, gel once each night.

Brands:
- Potassium nitrate 5%, fluoride toothpaste; Fludent-KF, Sensodent-K
- Sodium fluoride 0.2% + Potassium nitrate 3% Gel; Senquel-AD. Sodium fluoride 0.1% + Zinc sulfate 0.025%; Hydentgel
- Sodium fluoride 0.2% Rinse; fludent-M, Sensodent-F.
- Do not swallow/rinse paste or gel.

IRON

Uses: Treatment of microcytic hypochromic anemia, supplement in low birth weight babies, breast fed infants.

Dosage:
- RDA: 5–10 mg/day of elemental iron
- Prophylaxis: PO—1–2 mg/kg/day of elemental iron (maximum: 15 mg/day)

Deficiency:
- PO: 3–6 mg/kg/day of elemental iron in two divided doses
- IM, IV (for iron dextran in children >15 kg): Total dose (mL) = 0.0442 × (desired Hb - actual Hb) × lean body weight (kg) + (0.26 × lean body weight in kg). Give in divided doses.

Brands:
- 100 mg tablet; 50 mg/5 mL syrup; 50 mg/mL drops, elemental iron; Feritin, Feritone, Ferium, Ferose. 80 mg/5 mL pediatric syrup; 25 mg/mL elemental iron drops; Tonoferon. 60 mg/5 mL syrup; 20 mg/mL elemental iron drops; Ferrochelate. 25 and 50 mg tablet; 25 mg/5 mL elemental iron in syrup; Rarecap.
- May cause gastrointestinal (GI) irritation, nausea, diarrhea, dark stools, constipation, urine discoloration, teeth staining. Avoid in patient requiring frequent blood transfusion. When using for iron deficiency anemia, treat for additional 3–4 months after Hb return to normal in order to replenish total body iron stores.

ZINC

Uses: Prevention and treatment of zinc deficiency, maintenance treatment of Wilson's disease (zinc acetate), acrodermatitis enteropathica, anemia; increase wound healing in deficiency states, diarrhea.

Dosage:
- RDA: <1 year: 5 mg/day; 1–10 years: 10 mg/day; >10 years: 15 mg/day of elemental zinc.

Deficiency: PO—0.5–1 mg/kg/day in 2–3 divided doses
- Acrodermatitis enteropathica: 6 mg/kg/day.
- Acute diarrhea: <6 months: 10 mg/day as a single dose; >6 months: 20 mg/day as a single dose for 14 days.
- Wilsons disease: 2–12 years: 25 mg/day; 12–18 years: 50 mg/day; 2–4 times/day.

Brands: 20 mg/5 mL syrup; Zinconia, Emzinc. 10 mg tablet; Zinconia, Emzinc.
- Zinc may decrease penicillamine, quinolone, and tetracycline absorption. Iron and H_2 blockers decrease zinc absorption.

MAGNESIUM AND POTASSIUM

Refer Chapter 32 'Supplements and Fluid Replacements'.

Nutritional Supplements

chapter 37

ALFACALCIDOL

Uses: Treatment of hypocalcemia, renal rickets, vitamin D deficiency rickets, osteomalacia, hypoparathyroidism.

Dosage: PO
- Premature neonates and infants: 0.05–0.1 µg/kg/day
- Children: <20 kg: 0.05 µg/kg daily; >20 kg: 1.0 µg/day.

Brands: Alfacalcidol 0.25 µg + Calcium 200 mg tablet; Alcalci, Alfaarocal. 0.25, 1 µg cap; Alphadol. Alfacol, Alfarich.

CALCIUM PHOSPHATE

Uses: Strong bone growth, inhibits the progression of enamel subsurface lesions and prevents calcium deficiency in children.

Dosage: PO—children—5 mL syrup after meals.

Brands: 200 mL syrup: Ostocalcium B_{12} syrup B/F; each 5 mL contains Vitamin D_3 200 IU, vitamin B_{12}: 2.5 mg; calcium: 82 mg. Ostocalcium B_{12} syrup L/L; each 5 mL contains vitamin D_3 200 IU, vitamin B_{12} and calcium: 82 mg. Ostocalcium tablet; vitamin D_3 400 IU, 2.5 mg; tribasic calcium phosphate IP 0.323 g (equivalent to 125 mg of calcium).

CARNITINE

Uses: Treatment of carnitine deficiency, to improve IV fat emulsions utilization by premature neonates, cardiomyopathy, myopathy, long-term hemodialysis, Rett syndrome, supplement during valproate therapy.

Dosage:
- Premature neonates—IV: 10–20 mg/kg/day in parenteral nutrition solution

- Children: PO, IV—50–100 mg/kg/day in divided doses (maximum: 3 g/day PO and 1 g/dose for IV).

Brands: 330 and 500 mg tablet; 500 mg/5 mL syrup; 200 mg/mL injection; Carnitor. 500 mg/2.5 mL; 1 g/5 mL injection, Carnit.

FAT EMULSION

Uses: Source of calories and essential fatty acids for patients requiring parenteral nutrition for prolonged duration.

Dosage: IV
- Premature infants: Starting dose of 0.25–0.5 g/kg/day, increase by 0.25 g/kg/day to a maximum of 3 g/kg/day
- Infant and children: Starting dose of 0.5–1 g/kg/day, increase by 0.5 g/kg/day to a maximum of 4 g/kg/day.

Administration: Maximum rate of infusion in neonates is 0.15 g/kg/h or 0.75 mL/kg/h of 20% solution. In infants and children, it is 0.25 g/kg/h or 1.25 mL/kg/h of 20% solution. Heparin may be added in a dose of 1–2 units/mL.
- Fat calories should not exceed 60% of the total daily calories. 10% = 1.1 kcal/mL and 20% = 2 kcal/mL.

Brands: Intralipid IV: Contain soybean oil 100 mg/mL (10%) or 200 mg/mL (20%) + Fractioned egg phospholipid 12 g + Glycerol 22.5 g/100 mL. 10% in 100 and 500 mL bottle and 20% in 100 and 250 mL bottle.

MEDIUM CHAIN TRIGLYCERIDES (MCT OIL)

Uses: Nutritional supplement in infants for those who cannot digest long chain fats, induce ketosis as a prevention for seizures.

Doses:
- Infants: Start at 0.5 mL with every other feeding, then increase with every feeding
- Children (for seizures): About 40 mL with each meal or 50–70% of total calories.

Brands: Simyl MCT oil by FDC.
- May cause sedation, narcosis, ketosis, diarrhea.

Pituitary Hormones

chapter 38

ADRENOCORTICOTROPIN HORMONE (ACTH)

Uses: Infantile spasms, as immunosuppressant, severe muscle weakness in myasthenia gravis, west syndrome.

Dosage:
- Infantile spasms: IM, SC—initial dose of 20 units/day for 2 weeks if required effect occur then taper and discontinue over 1 week, if not responding increase to 30 units/day for 2 weeks sand then taper and discontinue over 1 week.
- Immunosuppression: IV, IM, SC—0.8 unit/kg/day divided q 12–24 hr.

Brands: 60 units/mL injection; Acton Prolongatum. 40 and 80 units/mL injection; Corticotrophin.

- May cause hypertension (HT), acne, Cushing's syndrome, sodium and water retention, hypokalemia. Do not stop abruptly.

DESMOPRESSIN

Uses: Primary nocturnal enuresis, diabetes insipidus.

Dosage:
- Diabetes insipidus: PO: 0.05 mg starting dose and titrate to effect to maximum of 0.8 mg/day. Intranasal: 5–30 µg/day in divided doses SC, IV: 2–5 µg/day in divided doses.
- Enuresis: >6 years of age; intranasal: 20 µg/day as starting dose can be increased up to 40 µg. PO: 0.05–0.1 mg at bedtime.

Brands: 0.1, 0.2 mg tablet; 4 µg/mL injection; Minirin. Nasal spray (10 µg/spray) D-Void, Minirin.

- Avoid intranasal use in patient of nasal edema, discharge, atopic rhinitis, obstruction. May cause facial flushing, tachycardia, headache, dizziness, hyponatremia.

GONADOTROPIN RELEASING HORMONE (GnRH)

Uses: Precocious puberty.

Dosage: Deep IM—3.75 mg q 4 weeks.

OCTREOTIDE

Uses: Hyperinsulinemia (if glucagon, diazoxide, and chlorthiazide fail), esophageal/gastric varices bleed, growth hormone excess.

Dosage:
- Hyperinsulinemia: SC—2–10 µg/kg/day divided q 12 hr and increased up to 40 µg/kg/day depending on response.
- Varices: IV infusion—1 µg/kg/hour initially, may be increased to 3 µg/kg/hour till bleeding is controlled, Then taper over 24 hours to avoid rebound bleeding.

Brands: 0.1 mg/mL ampoules; Octride, Sandostatin.
- For IV use dilute in normal saline (NS) to a ratio of not <1:1 and prepared solution should be used within 8 hours.

SOMATROPIN (GROWTH HORMONE)

Uses: Growth failure due to inadequate growth hormone secretion, chronic renal failure, short stature in Turner syndrome, Prader-Willi syndrome.

Dosage: IM, SC—0.06–0.16 IU/kg, 3 times/week.

Brands: 4, 12, 16 IU/vial; Genotropin. 4, 16, 18, and 36 IU/vial; Humatrope.
- May cause headache, intracranial hypertension with papilloedema, local lipoatrophy, reversible hypothyroidism.

VASOPRESSIN

Refer Chapter 26 'Cardiac Shocks and Failures'.

Plasma Volume Expanders

chapter 39

Plasma volume expanders are the agents that have high molecular weight and boost the plasma volume by increasing the osmotic pressure. These provide volume to the circulatory system and are used for fluid replacement.

ALBUMIN

Uses: Hypovolemia, plasma volume expansion and maintenance of cardiac output, hypoproteinemia, neonatal jaundice, cerebral edema, nephrotic syndrome.

Dosage:
- Hypoproteinemia: 0.5g/kg/dose, may be repeated q1–2 days
- Hypovolemia: 0.5 g/kg/dose, may be repeated as needed (maximum 1 g/kg/day in neonates and 6 g/kg/day in children).

Brands:
- 20% human albumin in 50 mL and 100 mL bottles; Albudac, Albumeon, Albupan
- 5% human albumin in 100 mL bottle; Sii Human Albumin
- 25% human albumin in 50 and 100 mL bottles; Albudac.

Administration: Rapid infusion may result in vascular overload. Rate of infusion should be 2–4 mL/min of 5% and 1 mL/min of 25% albumin. Albumin 5% should be used for hypovolemic patients and 25% should be used for patient with fluid or sodium restriction. Use lowest possible concentration in neonates.

DEXTRAN

Uses: Fluid replacement and blood volume expander in shock or impending shock; dextran 40 may be used for prophylaxis of venous thrombosis and pulmonary embolism.

Dosage: Dose and infusion rate must be individualized and be calculated depending upon the patient's fluid status. Total dose on day 1 is 20 mL/kg, second day onward it is 10 mL/kg/day and do not use for >5 days.

Brands: Dextran 40, 10% in normal saline (NS) or in 5% dextrose; Rallidex, Microspan-40. Dextran 70, 6% in NS or in 5% dextrose; Lamodex-70.

Contraindicated in chronic heart failure (CHF), renal failure, hypervolemia, thrombocytopenia, bleeding disorder; keep ready epinephrine and antihistamines to treat any anaphylactic reactions.

GELATIN

Uses: Hypovolemic shock, burns, cardiopulmonary bypass surgery.

Dosage: IV
- In hypovolemic shock 10–20 mL/kg bolus as rapidly as possible. Repeat as necessary. In trauma these requirements may increase upto 40 mL/kg. At this level, replacement with whole blood should be considered.

Brands: 500 mL infusion (contains degraded gelatin, electrolytes, distilled water, polypeptides); Haemaccel.

Scabicidal Agents

chapter 40

SCABICIDAL AGENTS

Scabicidal agents should be applied from head to toe in children for 2–3 days followed by thorough bath after 8–12 hours of application. Avoid contact with eyes, face, mucous membranes, urethral meatus and do not apply to inflamed or raw skin. These agents are also helpful in treatment of pediculosis. Course can be repeated after 7–10 days if required. Give antibiotic for secondary infection and also antipruritic agents if required.

BENZYL BENZOATE

Uses: Scabies, pediculosis.

Dosage:
- Scabies: Apply emulsion to entire body except head and face. Allow the medicine to remain on body for 24 hours, then thouroughly wash the body with warm water and soap. Treatment may need to be repeated for sever infestation.
- Pediculosis: Apply enough medicine to thoroughly wet the dry hair and scalp for 24 hours, then wash with warm water and soap. After rinsing and drying use fine comb to remove any remaining nits or nit shells.

Brands: 25% lotion; Benzyl benzoate.

CROTAMITON

Uses: Scabies, pruritis.

Dosge: Topical—after having a warm bath and dried well. Medicine should be rubbed to the entire body surface excluding face and scalp.

The application should be repeated once daily preferably in the evening for total 3–5 days.

Brands: 10% cream and lotion; Crotorax.

GAMMA BENZENE HEXACHLORIDE

Uses: Scabies, pediculosis.

Dosage:
- Scabies: Apply to whole body surface below neck. Scrub bath after 12–24 hours. If required one more application may be repeated after a week.
- Pediculosis: Massage scalp with emulsion at night and cover with a piece of cloth. Following morning, head bath should be taken ensuring that medication does not enter eyes. Comb the hair with fine comb after drying the hair.

Brands: 1% lotion; Scaboma, Welscab. 1% emulsion; Ascabiol.

PERMETHRIN

Uses: Scabies, Pediculosis.

Dosage:
- Scabies: Cream–single topical application: If required second application can be given after 7 days. Apply to whole body excluding head. Wash aff after 8–12 hours.
- Pediculosis: Apply to clean damp hair, leave on for 10 minutes rinse and dry. Then comb with fine comb.

Brands: 5% cream; Clerkin, Permarid, Permite. 5% lotion; Permisol, Scabitol-p.

Skeletal Muscle Relaxants

chapter 41

BACLOFEN

Uses: Treatment of cerebral spasticity, neurodegenerative conditions, spinal cord lesions spasticity, trigeminal neuralgia.

Dosage: PO
- Initial dose: 1–12 years: 2.5 mg BD; 12–18 years, 5 mg BD
- Maintenance dose: 1–2 years: 5 mg TDS; 2–6 years: 10 mg TDS; 6–10 years: 20 mg TDS.

Brands: 10 and 25 mg tablet; Liofen, Lioresol, Riclofen. 50 mg injection; Liofen.

- When used along with benzodiazepines, opiates, tricyclic antidepressants, increased central nervous system (CNS) depression is seen
- Avoid abrupt withdrawl, it should be gradual over 1–2 weeks.

BOTULINUM A TOXIN (HEMAGGLUTININ COMPLEX)

Uses: Equinus foot deformity due to spasticity in cerebral palsy (CP) patients in approximately 2 years of age. Spasticity of other muscle in CP patients, spasmodic torticolis in adolescents, blepharospasm in adolescents, hemifacial spasm in adolescents, hyperhydrosis of axilla.

Dosage: IM
- Cerebal palsy: Total dose per sitting is 4 units/day. Total dose is divided equally between the involved muscles. Dose should not be repeated within 2 months.
- Blepharospasm: Initially, 1.25–2.5 units injected into the medial and lateral orbicularis occuli of the upper lid and the lateral orbicularis

occuli of lower lid. Subsequently dose may be increased up to maximum of 25 units/eye.
- Hemifacial spasm: Treat as for unilateral blepharospasm (as above). Inject other affected muscles as needed.
- Cervical dystonia: Tailor dosing to individual patient based on the head and neck position, location of pain, muscle hypertrophy, body weight and response. Do not inject sternocleidomastoid muscle bilaterally. Maximum total dose should not be >200 units.
- Hyperhidrosis of axilla: Inject 50 units intradermally to each axilla, evenly distributed to multiple sites 1–2 cm apart.

Brands: 100 units vial; Botox.
- Should only be used in hospital settings by persons appropriately trained for the use.
- Reconstitute with 0.9% normal saline (NS) without preservative and should be used within 24 hours.

CHLORZOXAZONE

Uses: Symptomatic treatment of muscle spasm and pain.

Dosage: PO—20 mg/kg/day in 3–4 divided doses.

Brands: Chlorzoxazone + Paracetamol (PCM): 250 + 300 mg tablet; Duodil, Myospaz, Parafon.
- May color urine orange or red, fever, rash, anorexia, hepatitis, drowsiness are the common side effects.

DANTROLENE

Uses: Treatment of spasticity associated with upper motor neuron (UMN) lesions (spinal cord injury, stroke, CP), malignant hyperthermia.

Dosage: PO
- Spasticity: Initial, 0.5 mg/kg/dose twice daily, can be increased weekly upto a maximum of 3 mg/kg/dose.
- Malignant hyperthermia: IV bolus—1 mg/kg as single dose repeated as required at 5–10 minutes intervals to maximum cumulative dose of 10 mg/kg.

Brands: 25, 50, 100 mg capsule; Dantrium. 20 mg injection; Dantrium.

METHOCARBAMOL

Uses: Supportive therapy in tetanus, muscle spasm associated with acute painful musculoskeletal condition.

Dosage: IV—tetanus: 15 mg/kg/dose q 6 hr for 3 days only.

Brands: 100 mg/mL injection; Robinax. Methacarbamol + PCM: 400 + 325 mg tablet; Flexinol, Neuromol-MR.

- May cause hypotension, bradycardia, drowsiness, headache, nausea.

Skin/Acne Drugs

chapter 42

ADAPALENE

Uses: Acne.

Dosage: Applied topically at bedtime, wash and dry the application area before application.

Brands: 0.1% gel; Aclene, Adapen, Adaple.

- Avoid application over eyes, lips, angles of nose, and mucous membrane
- Avoid exposure to sunlight
- Do not use with other drugs with similar action.

AZELAIC ACID

Uses: Acne.

Dosage: Topically; wash the affected area with water then apply a thin layer initially once daily, then gradually increase to twice daily. Should not be used for >6 months.

Brands: 10 and 20% cream; Aziderm.

- Avoid contact with eyes and lips.

BENZOYL PEROXIDE

Uses: Acne.

Dosage:
- Topically: Apply a thin layer 1–2 times per day
- Clean the affected area with clean water before application.

Brands: 2.5% gel; Benzac AC, Persol, Pernox.

Side effect: Transient redness and skin peeling may occur.

CALAMINE LOTION

Uses: Pruritus.

Dosage: Apply to external affected area as needed.

Brands: 8% Calamine + Diphenhydramine lotion; Caladryl.

CLOBETASONE

For details *refer* Chapter 29 'Corticosteroids'.

TRETINOIN

Uses: Acne.

Dosage: Topically—wash the affected area thoroughly with water before appliction. Apply a thin layer 1–2 times/day.

Brands: 0.05% cream; Retino-A. 0.025, 0.05, 0.1% gel; A-Ret.

- Cream is recommended for dry or fair skin, gel for oily or dark skin. Avoid contact with eyes, nostrils, and mucous membranes. Minimize exposure to sunlight.

Sympathomimetics

chapter 43

ADRENALINE/EPINEPHRINE

Uses: Cardiac arrest, bronchospasm, anaphylactic reaction.

Dosages:
- Neonates: IV, intratracheal; 0.01–0.03 mg/kg q 3–5 minutes as needed (0.1–0.3 mL/kg of 1:10,000 solution)
- Infants and children:
  - SC: 0.01 mg/kg (0.01 mL/kg of 1:1000 solution)
  - IV: 0.01 mg/kg (0.1 mL/kg of 1:10,000 solution); maximum: 1 mg, may be repeated q 3–5 minutes as needed
- Intratracheal: 0.1 mg/kg (0.1 mL/kg of 1:1,000 solution); maximum: 0.2 mL/kg
- Continuous infusion: 0.1–1 µg/kg/min
- Inhalation: 0.1 mL/kg of 1:10,000 solution by nebulizer diluted in 3 mL of normal saline (NS).

Brands: 1 mg/mL of 1:1,000 dilution injection; Adrenaline, Enatrate, Vasocon.
- May cause pallor, tachycardia, hypertension (HT), headache, tremor, nausea, etc.
- Incompatible with sodium bicarbonate.

DOBUTAMINE

Uses: Treatment of hypotension persisting after adequate fluid volume replacement.

Dosage: 5–20 µg/kg/min as continuous infusion and titrate to response (maximum: 40 µg/kg/min).

Brands: 250 mg/vial; Cardiforce, Cardiject, Dobustat.
- Diluted in NS or dextrose, maximum recommended concentration is 5,000 µg/mL (5 mg/mL). May cause ectopics, tachycardia, tachyarrhythmias, leg cramps, paresthesias. Do not administer via umbilical arterial catheter in neonates.

DOPAMINE

Uses: Treatment of shock and hypotension unresponsive to adequate fluid volume replacement.

Dosage: 1–20 µg/kg/min continuous infusion, titrate to desired response (maximum: 20 µg in neonates and 50 µg/kg/min in infants and children).

Brands: 40 mg/mL injection; Dopacard, Dopa-plus, Dopar.
- If dose >30 µg/kg/min is required then direct acting agents such as epinephrine and norepinephrine may be more beneficial. Maximum concentration allowed for IV use 3,200 µg/mL. May cause ectopics, tachycardia, vasoconstriction, ventricular arrhythmias, decrease during output in high doses. Do not administer via umbilical arterial catheter in neonates.

EPHEDRINE

Uses: Nasal congestion.

Dosage: 2 drops in each nostril 2–3 times/day.

Brands: Ephedrine 0.75% and 0.5% + Menthol 0.5% + Camphor 0.5% + Eucalyptol 0.5% + Castor oil 0.5%; Drop Endrine and Endrine mild.

NOREPINEPHRINE

Uses: As dopamine

Dosage: 0.05–0.1 µg/kg/min, titrate to required effect (maximum: 2 µg/kg/min).

Brands: 1 mg/mL base injection; Adrenor, Levonor, Norad.
- May cause arrhythmias, bradycardia, tachycardia, organ ischemia due to vasoconstriction, etc.

OXYMETAZOLINE

Uses: Symptomatic relief of nasal congestion.

Dosage:
- 2–12 years: 0.025%, 2–3 drop 3 times/day
- >12 years: 0.05%, 2–3 drop 3 times/day.

Brands: 0.025 and 0.05% nasal drop; Nasivion and Sinarest.

PHENYLEPHRINE

Uses: Symptomatic relief of nasal and nasopharyngeal mucosal congestion, as a mydriatic in ophthalmic procedure.

Dosage: Nasal congestion—1–2 drop/nostril q 6 hr, should not be used for >5 days. Ophthalmic procedure: 1 drop 15–30 minutes before procedure.

Brands: 0.25% nasal drop; Andre and Fenox. 5% eye drop; Efrosyn, Fenilefrina.

- Causes rebound congestion on prolonged nasal use.

PSEUDOEPHEDRINE

Refer Chapter 13 'Antihistamines'.

XYLOMETAZOLINE

Uses: Symptomatic relief of nasal congestion.

Dosage:
- 2–12 years: 2–3 drop of 0.05% solution q 8 hr
- >12 years: 2–3 drop of 0.1% solution q 8 hr.

Brands: 0.05 and 0.1% pediatric and adult nose drop; Decon, Otrivin.

Thyroid and Antithyroid Agents

chapter 44

CARBIMAZOLE

Uses: Hyperthyroidism, in thyrotoxicosis prior to thyroidectomy.

Dosage: PO—1–2 mg/kg/day divided q 8 hr.

Brands: 5, 10 and 20 mg tablet; Neo-Mercazole, Thyrocab.

- May cause hypothyroidism, gastrointestinal (GI) disturbances, rash, agranulocytosis.

LIOTHYRONINE

Uses: Replacement therapy in congenital or acquired hypothyroidism.

Dosage: PO—initial dose of 5 µg/day, may be increased by 5 µg q 3 days to a maximum of 20 µg/day for <1 year; 50 µg/day for 1–3 years and 75 µg/day for >3 years.

Brands: 20 µg tablet; Tetroxin. 20 µg injection; Triiodothyronine.

- May cause palpitations, arrhythmias, hypertension (HT), weight loss, tremor, diaphoresis, insomnia.

PROPYLTHIOURACIL

Uses: Hyperthyroidism, thyrotoxic crisis.

Dosage: PO—5–7 mg/kg/day divided q 8 hr and titrate to the required effect. Maintenance dose usually begins after 2 months and it is 1/3 to 2/3 of the initial dose, given divided q 8–12 hr.

Brand: 50 mg tablet; Propylthiouracil (PTU).

THYROXINE

Uses: As liothyronine.

Dosage: PO—0–6 months: 10–15 µg/kg; 6–12 months: 6–8 µg/kg; 1–5 years: 5–6 µg/kg; 6–12 years: 4–5 µg/kg; >12 years: 2–3 µg/kg.

Brands: 25 and 50 µg tablet; Thyrochek, Thyrox, Thyronorm. 100 µg tablet; Eltroxin, Roxin.

Vaccines

BACILLUS CALMETTE-GUÉRIN (BCG)

Live attenuated vaccine of bovine strain, contains 0.1–0.4 million mycobacteria.

Uses: Tuberculosis and leprosy prevention.

Dosage: Given 0.1 mL intradermal, use within 4 hours of reconstitution, given from birth to 60 days. Reconstitute with normal saline (NS) and administer over the middle of the left deltoid area using a 26/27 G needle. Do not use antiseptic for cleansing the injection site.

Brands: 10 dose/vial by Aventis and Serum.

DIPHTHERIA, PERTUSSIS, AND TETANUS (DPT)

Available as either whole cell or highly purified acellular component vaccine. Contain diphtheria toxoid >20 to <30 limit of flocculation (Lf), toxoid vaccine (TT) >5 to <40 Lf and *B. pertussis* 20,000 million killed bacteria per dose. Acellular vaccine has lower incidence of side effects. Also available in combination with *Haemophilus influenzae* type b (Hib), inactivated polio vaccine (IPV) and hepatitis-B.

Uses: Diptheria and tetanus prophylaxis, whooping cough prophylaxis.

Dosage: Primary doses at 6, 10, 14 weeks and booster at 18 months and 4–5 years. Given 0.5 mL deep IM.

Brands: Triple antigen (whole cell); single and multidose vial.

DIPHTHERIA-TETANUS (DT)

Uses: Diptheria and tetanus prophylaxis.

Dosage: Indicated in children, where pertussis component is contraindicated. Contain diphtheria toxoid 20–30 Lf and TT 5–25 Lf, given 0.5 mL IM at 10 and 16 years of age.

Brands: Dual antigen; single and multidose vial.

HEPATITIS-B

Hepatitis B is a purified surface antigen vaccine, either genetically engineered or plasma derived. Available in combination with Hib, DPT and IPV.

Uses: Hepatitis-B prophylaxis.

Dosage: Contain 10 μg/0.5 mL, given IM. Primary doses at birth, 6, 14 week or 6, 10, 14 weeks or 0, 1, 6 months. 10 μg up to 18 years and 20 μg in older children and high-risk individuals.

Postexposure prophylaxis may require 4 doses at 0, 1, 2 months and 1 year (accelerated) or 0, 7, 21 days and 1 year (superaccelerated).

Brands: Bevac, Engerix-B, Genevac-B, single and multidose vial.

HEPATITIS-A

Available as inactivated and live attenuated forms.

Uses: Hepatitis-A prophylaxis in high-risk group, travelers, chronic liver disease, etc.

Dosage: Given after 1 year of age in two primary doses given at 1 year intervals.

Brands: Havrix; 720 ELISA units/0.5 mL and 1440 ELISA units/1 mL of HM-175 in activated antigen. Avaxim; 80U/0.5 mL and 160U/1 mL of inactivated GBM strain. Biovac-A; 6.5 LgCCID50/1 mL of H_2 attenuated strain. Havrix and Avaxim given IM and Biovac-A SC.

HAEMOPHILUS INFLUENZAE TYPE-B CONJUGATE

Conjugate of purified capsular polysaccharide to either diphtheria or tetanus toxoid (PRP-D, PRP-T). Available in combination with DPT, IPV and hepatitis-B.

Uses: *Haemophilus influenzae* type-B invasive disease prophylaxis, asplenia, immunocompromised children.

Dosage: Given IM 0.5 mL in 3 doses when started below 6 months, 2 doses between 6 and 12 months and 1 dose between 12 and 15 months. Booster between 15–18 months. Between 18 months and 5 years single primary dose. Asplenia patient require only single dose.

Brands: Hiberix, Act-HIB, Novohib; 10 μg of PRP-T/0.5 mL. Hibtitre, Vaxemhib; 10 μg of PRP-D/0.5 mL.

HUMAN PAPILLOMAVIRUS VACCINE (HPV)

Uses: Prevention of persistent human papilloma virus infection and sequelly including cervical cancer, vulvar cancer and vaginal cancer caused by HPV.

Dosage:
- Gardesil: It is a mixture of L1 protiens of HPV serotypes 16, 18, 6 and 11.
- Cervarix: It is a bivalent vaccine containing L1 proteins of HPV serotypes 16 and 18.
- The vaccine is given IM over deltoid region in 3 doses to women between 14 and 46 years (gardesil 0,2 and 6 months; cervarix 0,1 6 months). During 9–14 years, two doses are recommended at 0,6 months.

Brands: Inj; Cervarix, Gardasil.

INFLUENZA VIRUS VACCINE

Uses: Prophylaxis against influenza infection in—bronchopulmonary dysplasia, asthma, chronic heart disease, cyanotic congenital heart disease, chronic renal failure, diabetes mellitus, asplenia, Down's syndrome.

Dosage: Influenza virus vaccine is an inactivated vaccine containing hemagglutinin of each of three recommended strains (influenza-A, H1N1, H3N1, and influenza-B). Given IM, children between 6 month 3 year 0.25 mL single dose if previously vaccinated otherwise 2 doses at 4 weeks interval, if >3 years dose is 0.5 mL. Revaccinate every year with strain adjusted vaccine.

Brands: Injection; Agrippal, FluQuadri, Fluarix, Influgen.

INACTIVATED POLIO VACCINE

Uses: Poliomyelitis prophylaxis.

Dosage: Inactivated polio vaccine is an inactivated salk strain vaccine. Given IM, 3 primary doses at 6, 10, 14 weeks or 8, 12, 16 weeks; booster at 15 month (at an interval of 6 months from 3rd dose). Also available in combination with HIB, DPT and hepatitis-B.

Brands: Imovax, Polprotec; contain type 1 >40 DU + type 2 >08 DU + type 3 >32 DU/0.5 mL.

JAPANESE ENCEPHALITIS

Uses: Japanese encephalitis prophylaxis in children >1 year of age.

Dosage: Jeev is given IM in a dose of 3 µg/dose for children 1–3 years and 6 µg/dose in older children; as 2 primary doses on day 0 and 28.
- Jenvac is given IM, 0.5 mL after the age of 1 year as a single dose.

Brands: Injection; Jeev and Jenvac.

MEASLES

Uses: Measles prophylaxis.

Dose: Live attenuated Edmonston-Zagreb strain vaccine. Given subcutaneous (SC) at 9 months of completed age as single dose. In case of an outbreak; however, the vaccine may be given to infants as young as 6 months of age. Should be used within 4 hours of reconstitution.

Brands: M-VAC; 1,000 CCID50/0.5 mL.

MEASLES, MUMPS AND RUBELLA (MMR)

Live attenuated vaccine.

Uses: Prophylaxis against measles, mumps and rubella.

Dose: Given SC in 2 doses at the age of 9 months and 15–18 months of age. Third dose may be given at 4–6 year of age.

Brands: Tresivac; Measles E-Z strain >1,000 CCID50 + Mumps L-Z strain >5,000 CCID50 + Rubella RA 27/3 strain >1,000 CCID50 per 0.5 mL. Injection Priorix; Measles Schwarz strain >1,000 CCID50 + Mumps RIT 4385 >1,000 CCID50 + Rubella RA 27/3 >1,000 CCID50/0.5 mL, injection.

MENINGOCOCCAL

An inactivated capsular polysaccharide vaccine.

Dose: Given IM in >2 years of age during an epidemic, single dose followed by booster every 2 years.

Brands: Mencevax injection; each 0.5 mL dose contain 50 µg of A, C, W and Y serotype. Meningococcal injection; each 0.5 mL dose contain 50 µg of A and C serotype.

ORAL POLIO VACCINE (OPV)

Uses: Poliomyelitis prophylaxis and eradication.

Dosage: Live-attenuated Sabin strain vaccine. Given PO 2 drops at birth. Following posteradication, bivalent oral polio vaccine is being used containing type-1 and type-3 polio strain.

Brands: OPV 20 dose vial by Haffkine and GSK, contain type 1 >10^6, type 3 >$10^{5.5}$ CCID50 per dose.

PNEUMOCOCCAL VACCINE

Uses: Pneumococcal invasive disease prophylaxis.

Dosage: Pneumococcal vaccine is a polysaccharide vaccine available in 13 and 23 valent forms. Recommended in >2 years, 23 valent is given 0.5 mL IM or SC single dose followed by booster after 3–5 years. For 13 valent primary doses are given at 6, 10, 14 weeks followed by booster at 12–15 months.

Brands: Pneumo-23, Pnu-Imune 23, 0.5 mL dose contain 25 µg of each serotype. Prevenar is a 13 valent and contain 2 µg of each serotype.

RABIES

Uses: Prophylaxis against rabies.
- Rabies vaccine is an inactivated tissue culture vaccine. Available as human diploid cell vaccine (HDCV), purified chick embryo vaccine (PCEV) and purified vero cell rabies vaccine (PVRV). Rabies immunoglobulin is recommended in all category 3 bites along with vaccine.

Dosage: Given IM, pre-exposure prophylaxis consist of 3 doses at 0, 7 and 28 days and postexposure schedule is 0, 3, 7, 14, 28, and 90 days. If a child is vaccinated previously within 3 years, for postexposure prophylaxis only 2 doses on day 0 and 3 are given. The vaccine should not be given in the gluteal region as the antibody response may be reduced.

Brands: Rabipur injection; (PCEV) 0.5 mL/dose; Rabivax injection; (HDCV) 0.5 mL/dose. Verorab injection; (PVRV) 0.5 mL/dose.

ROTAVIRUS VACCINE

Uses: Rotavirus gastroenteritis prophylaxis.

Dosage: Rotarix is a live-attenuated human rotavirus RIX4414 strain vaccine containing not <106 CCID50. Given PO, two doses at 4 weeks interval starting from 6 weeks of age onwards.
- RotaTeq RV-5 is a human bovine pentavalent vaccine containing 5 rotavirus strains and is available in liquid ready to use form. Rotavac is attenuated 116E rotavirus Indian strain. These two vaccines are given in 3 doses 4 weeks apart starting from 6 weeks onwards. All the doses should be completed before 32 weeks of age.

Brands: Rotarix; single dose 1 mL. Rota Teq, Rotavac.

RUBELLA

Uses: Rubella infection prophylaxis.

Dosage: Vaccine contain live-attenuated rubella virus Wistar RA 27/3 strain. Dose is 0.5 mL SC over deltoid region.

Brands: Injection; R-vac single dose vial.

TETANUS AND DIPHTHERIA (TD)

Uses: Tetanus and diphtheria prophylaxis.

Dosage: TD is a low dose diphtheria vaccine combined with tetanus toxoid, recommended in >7 years of age and routinely at 10 and 16 years; should replace TT at 10 and 16 years. Given 0.5 mL IM.

Brands: TD Vac injection; Contain diphtheria toxoid <5 Lf and TT >5 Lf/dose.

TETANUS, DIPHTHERIA, PERTUSSIS (TDAP)

Uses: Tetanus, diphtheria, and whooping cough prophylaxis.

Dosage: Vaccine contain diphtheria toxoid 2 Lf and tetanus toxoid 5 Lf and acellular pertusis 2.5–8 µg. Indicated for adolescents and adults for pertusis vaccination. Dose is 0.5 mL IM single dose.

Brands: Injection; Boostrix and Adacel.

TYPHOID

Typhoid vaccine is a purified Vi capsular polysaccharide vaccine. Given IM after 2 years of age and booster every 3 years. IAP recommends the use of new Vi conjugate vaccine below 1 year of age, preferably between 9 and 12 months

Brands: Enteroshield, Typbar-TCV, Zyvac-TCV injection; Contain 25 µg of *Salmonella* type 2 (Vi antigen).

TETANUS (TT)

Uses: Active protection for tetanus, routine immunization of infants and children at 10 years, wounds if last tetanus vaccine was given year ago.

Dosage: TT is an alum-precipitated toxoid vaccine, contain 5–25 Lf of toxoid. Given 0.5 mL IM.

Brand: Injection; Bett single dose ampule.

VARICELLA/CHICKEN POX VACCINE

Uses: Chickenpox active prophylaxis, herpes zoster prophylaxis, renal transplant candidate, leukemia in remission, household contacts of immunocompromised children.

Dosage: Live-attenuated Oka strain vaccine. Given SC, single dose in 1–13 years and 2 doses in >13 years with a gap of 4 weeks.

Brands: Varivax injection—contain ≥2,000 PFU/dose. Okavax injection; contain ≥1,000 PFU.

YELLOW FEVER

Uses: Yellow fever prophylaxis to children >9 months for travelers to endemic area.

Dosage: Is a live attenuated vaccine with >100 units of virus count/0.5 ml. Given IM or SC as a single dose after 1 year of age.

Brand: Injection; Stamaril.

Vasodilators

chapter 46

NITROGLYCERIN

Uses: Shock, portal hypertension, congestive heart failure (CHF), hypertensive emergencies.

Dosage: In children by continuous infusion. Initial: 0.25–0.5 µg/kg/minute; titrate by 0.5–1 µg/kg/min q 3–5 min to maximum of 5 -10 µg/kg/min.

Brands: 5 mg/mL injection; NIG, Nitrocin, Nitroject.
- For IV use dilute in D-5% or normal saline (NS) to 50–100 µg/mL. Vasodilates veins more than arteries. May cause flushing, hypotension, reflex tachycardia, dizziness, headache.

TOLAZOLINE

Uses: Treatment of persistent pulmonary hypertension, improve pulmonary circulation in ventilated babies.

Dosage: Neonates—IV; 1–2 mg/kg loading dose followed by 0.2 mg/kg/h continuous infusion.
- May cause hypotension, tachycardia, increased respiratory and gastrointestinal (GI) secretions, GI bleed, flushing, pulmonary hemorrhage.

Captropil, Diazoxide, Enalapril, Hydralazine, Minoxidil, Nifedipine
Nitroprusside, Phenoxybenzamine, Phentolamine, Prazosin

For details of these drugs *Refer* **Chapter 14 'Antihypertensives'.**

Vitamins

chapter 47

BIOTIN

Uses: Nutritional biotin deficiency, primary biotinidase deficiency, propionic acidemias, holocarboxylase synthetase deficiency.

Dosage:
- Recommended dietary allowance (RDA): 10–200 μg/day
- Biotinidase deficiency propionic acidemias, holocarboxylase synthetase deficiency: 5–10 mg once daily
- Biotin deficiency: 5–20 mg once daily.

Brands: 5 mg tablet; H-Vit, Oltin.

CYANOCOBALAMIN/VITAMIN B_{12}

Uses: Megaloblastic anemia, nutritional supplement, increased B_{12} requirement due to hemorrhage, liver or kidney disease.

Dosage:
- RDA: 0.3–2μg/day
- Megaloblastic anemia: IM; 30–50 μg/day to total dose of 1,000–5,000 μg and then 100 μg per month
- Deficiency: 100 μg/day for 15 days then once or twice weekly for several month.

Brands: 1,000 μg vitamin B_{12} in 2 mL ampule along with vitamin B_1 and B_6; Bevidex, Macrabarin. 500, 1,000 μg tablet; Bigvin. 1,000 μg/mL injection; Citon.

- Severe hypokalemia may occur after conversion of megaloblastic anemia to normal erythropoiesis, so serum potassium level should be monitored.

FOLIC ACID

Uses: Megaloblastic and macrocytic anemia, tropical sprue, during phenytoin therapy, juvenile idiopathic arthritis.

Dosage:
- RDA: Neonates—6 months: 30 μg/day. 6 months–3 years: 50 μg/day. 4–6 years: 75 μg/day. 7–10 years: 100 μg/day. >11 years: 150 μg/day.
- Deficiency: 5 mg/day.

Brands: 5 mg tablet; Fol-5, Folet, Folium, Folvite.
- Large doses may mask the hematologic effect of B_{12} deficiency while allowing the neurologic complication due to deficiency to progress.

NIACIN/NICOTINIC ACID/VITAMIN B_3

Uses: Treatment of pellagra, dietary supplement, hyperlipidemia, long-term treatment of certain medications (such as isoniazid).

Dosage:
- RDA: 5–15 mg/day
- Pellagra: 50–100 mg/dose 3 times/day
- Hyperlipidemia: 10 mg/kg/day is maximum dose.

Brands: Nicotinic acid 5 mg + vitamin B_2 5 mg + vitamin B_6 1.5 mg + vitamin B_{12} 7 μg + niacinamide 45 mg + vitamin C 75 mg/5 mL Syrup; Beplex Forte. 375 mg and 500 mg tablet; Neasyn, Nialip.

PYRIDOXINE/VITAMIN B_6

Uses: Prevention and treatment of B_6 deficiency, pyridoxine-dependent seizures, sideroblastic anemia, treatment of drug-induced deficiency, e.g., isoniazid, cycloserine, hydralazine.

Dosage:
- RDA: 0.5–1.5 mg/day
- Pyridoxine-dependent seizures: PO, IV, IM—50–100 mg initial dose, maintenance dose: 50–100 mg/day, PO
- Dietary deficiency: 5–15 mg/day for 3–4 weeks then 2.5–5 mg/day
- Drug-induced neuritis: PO– for treatment 10–50 mg/day and for prophylaxis 1–2 mg/kg/day.

Brands: 40 mg tablet; Benadon. 100 mg tablet; B-Long, Pyricontin. 100 mg pyridoxine + B_1 + B_6 injection; Bevidox, Neurokem. Pyridoxine 3 mg + Nicotinamide 100 mg + Cyano-cobalamin 15 µg + Folic acid 1,500 µg + Chromium picolinate 250 µg + Selenium 100 µg per capsule; Cobadex. Cobadex-Z in addition contain elemental zinc 22.5 mg per capsule.

- Sensory neuropathy may occur after chronic administration of large doses and large IV doses may precipitate seizures.

RIBOFLAVIN/VITAMIN B_2

Uses: Prevention and treatment of riboflavin deficiency, glutaric acidemia type-1 and 2, congenital lactic acidosis.

Dosage:
- RDA: 0.5–1 mg/day
- Deficiency: 2.5–10 mg/day in divided doses.
- Metabolic disease: 50–150 mg every 12–24 hours

Brands: 20 mg tablet; Lipabol. 5 mg tablet; Riboflavin, Ribosina.

THIAMINE/VITAMIN B_1

Uses: Beriberi, Wernicke's encephalopathy, peripheral neuritis, congenital lactic acidosis, maple syrup urine disease (MSUD).

Dosage:
- RDA: 0.2–1 mg/day or 0.5 mg/1,000 kcal diet
- Beriberi: PO, IM, IV—10–30 mg/day for 2 week then 5–10 mg PO/day for 1 month
- Encephalopathy: IM, IV—100 mg/day until consuming a regular balanced diet.
- MSUD: PO—10–300 mg once daily.
- Congenital lactic acidosis: PO: 100–300 mg once daily.

Brands: 75 mg tablet; Benalgis. 100 mg tablet; Beneuron forte, Berin. Thiamine 10 mg + vitamin B_2 10 mg + vitamin B_{12} 15 µg + Folic acid 1500 µg + Calcium pantothenate 50 mg + vitamin C 150 mg, capsule; Glace-X. 100 mg/mL injection; Berin.

- Rapid IV administration may lead to cardiovascular collapse and death.

VITAMIN A

Uses: Treatment and prevention of vitamin A deficiency, supplementation in children with measles.

Dosage:
- RDA: 1,000–3,000 IU/day as per age
- Deficiency: PO– >1 year: 200,000 IU for 2 days and then 1–4 weeks later. 6–12 months: ½ of above dose and in <6 months 1/4 of the above dose and schedule. Parenteral dose is ½ of the PO dose.
- Prophylaxis in patient at risk (malnutrition, severe infection, recurrent diarrhea, pneumonia). In <1 year: 100,000 units and in >1 year: 200,000 units given PO every 4–6 months.

Brands: 50,000 units tablet; and capsule; 50,000 units/mL injection; Vitamin A.

- Hypervitaminosis A may occur with massive doses or with large doses given over long period and manifest as nausea, vomiting, drowsiness, papilledema, symptoms of raised intracranial pressure (ICP).

VITAMIN C/ASCORBIC ACID

Uses: Scurvy, urinary acidification, methemoglobinemia, congenital lactic acidosis.

Dosage:
- RDA: 30–50 mg/day
- Scurvy: 100–300 mg/day
- Urinary acidification: 500 mg q 6 hr
- To increase iron excretion during deferoxamine therapy: 100–200 mg/day.
- Metabolic indications: PO—100-400 mg/day.

Brands: 100 and 500 mg tablet; Celin, Cell-C. 100 mg/ mL drops; Cecon, Celin. 100 mg/mL injection; Redoxon, Tildoxon.

VITAMIN D/CHOLECALCIFEROL

Uses: Rickets, Vitamin-D deficiency, routine supplementation.

Dosage:
- RDA: very low birth weight (VLBW)—800 units/day. Birth–12 months: 400 units/day. >12 months: 600 units/day.
- Rickets: IM—5,000–50,000 units daily or one single dose of 3–600,000 units once in 3 weeks. If no signs of healing on skiagram after 3–9 week of therapy then repeat the dose and investigate for other causes.
- Deficiency: Premature neonates– 1,000 units/day. Term neonates and upto 6 months: 2,000 units/day. 6 months–12 years: 6,000 units/day. 12–18 years: 10,000 units/day.

Brands: 400 units/mL drops; Arbivit-3, Ultra-D3, Sunsip. 800 units/mL drops; Calcirol, Calcibest, Calshine-P. 3,00,000–6,00,000 units/sachet; Calcirol, D-rise, D-sol. 3,00,000 and 6,00,000 units/mL injection; Arachitol.

- High dose of vitamin D_3 given over long period may cause anorexia, vomiting, hypotonia, polydipsia, polyuria, hypercalcemia, hypercalciuria.

VITAMIN E/(α-TOCOPHEROL)

Uses: Vitamin E deficiency treatment and prevention, nocturnal muscle cramps, prevention of retinopathy and anemia of prematurity, chronic cholestasis, brochopulmonary dysplasia.

Dosage (1 mg = 1.5 units):
- Prevention: Neonates—5 units/day. Children—10–20 units/day.
- Cystic fibrosis: 100–400 unit/day.
- Beta-thalassemia: 750 unit/day.
- Sickle cell anemia: 450 unit/day.
- Deficiency: Neonates—25–50 units/day. Children–1 unit/kg/day.

Brands: 200 and 400 mg capsule; Evion, Evit, Tocofer, 50 mg/mL drops; Evion.

VITAMIN K

Uses: Nutritional supplement, hemorrhagic disease of the newborn, prevention and treatment of hypoprothrombinemia caused by vitamin K deficiency or anticoagulant-induced hypoprothrombinemia, hepatic failure, biliary atresia, malabsorption syndrome.

Dosage:
- HDN: 0.5 mg for preterm and 1 mg for term neonate within 1 hour of birth
- Biliary atresia and liver disease in neonates and babies: PO—1mg.
- Bleeding in patients due to vitamin K deficiency: SC/IV—2–10 mg.
- Bleeding disorders with mild abnormal coagulation: SC—1–5 mg.
- Children: IM, IV, SC—1–2 mg/dose. PO—2.5–5 mg/dose.

Brands: 10 mg/mL injection; Kapilin (vitamin K analog menaphthone) 1 mg/0.5 mL and 10 mg/mL injection; 10 mg tablet; Kenadion. (phytomenadione).
 – Not effective in hypoprothrombinemia due to severe liver disease and hereditary hypoprothrombinemia.

Miscellaneous Drugs

ALPRAZOLAM

Uses: Treatment of anxiety and panic disorder.

Dosage: PO—0.005–0.02 mg/kg/dose 3 times/day.

Brands: 0.25 and 0.5 mg tablet; Alprax, Alzolam, Restyl.

- Abrupt discontinuation may result in withdrawal symptoms. Safety not established in <18 years.

ATOMOXETINE

Uses: Attention deficit hyperactivity disorder.

Dosage: PO–children and adolescents: Initially 0.5 mg/kg/day may be increased after 3 days to a target dose of 1.2 mg/kg/day, given once or twice daily doses.

Brands: 18, 25 mg tablet; Attentrol, Axepta.

ATORVASTATIN

Uses: Hypercholesterolemia in patient not responding adequately to diet and other measures.

Dosage: PO–children >6 years: 10–40 mg/day once daily. Adjust dose as per lipid levels.

Brands: 10 and 20 mg tablet; Astin, Astorlip, Atorva, Lilo.

- May cause hepatitis, pancreatitis, gastritis, hyperglycemia.

AZATHIOPRINE

Uses: Adjunct with other agents in prevention of transplant rejection, as immunosuppressant in autoimmune diseases, such as Systemic lupus erythematosus (SLE), nephrotic syndrome, rheumatoid arthritis.

Dosage: PO, IV
- Transplantation: Initial 2–5 mg/kg/dose once daily and maintenance dose is 1–3 mg/kg/dose once daily
- Other condition: 1 mg/kg/dose once daily for 6–8 weeks.

Brands: 50 mg tablet; Azimune, Azoprine, Imuran. 100 mg/vial; Imuran.
- If used along with allopurinol reduce dose by 25–33%. Chronic immunosuppression increases risk of lymphoma and skin cancers. May cause irreversible bone marrow suppression.

CAFFEINE CITRATE

Uses: Idiopathic apnea of prematurity.

Dosage : Neonate; IV
- Loading dose: 10–20 mg/kg (5–10 mg/kg as caffeine base)
- Maintenance dose: 5 mg/kg/day (2.5 mg/kg/day as caffeine base) once daily, started 24 hours after the loading dose. Adjust maintenance dose based on patient response.

Brands : 20 mg/mL injection; Cafirate, Cafcit, Capnea. 20 mg/mL oral solution; Cafirate, Primicef.
- Give loading dose over at least 30 minutes and maintenance dose over 10 minutes diluted in D 5%.

CALAMINE

Uses: Pruritis.

Dosage: Apply to external affected area as needed.

Brands: 8% lotion; Caladry, Calapure.

CALCIUM POLYSTYRENE SULFONATE (ION EXCHANGE RESIN)

Uses: Hyperkalemia.

Dosage: Rectally and orally: 125–250 mg/kg 4 times daily. Not recommended in neonates. Give orally mixed with water, avoid mixing with fruit juices because of the high potassium content. For rectal use mix 1 g with 5–10 mL methylcellulose.

Brands: 15 g sachet; K-Bind.

CHARCOAL

Uses: Emergency treatment in poisoning by certain drugs and chemicals, in overdoses of certain drugs to enhance their excretion (phenobarbital, quinine, carbamazepine).

Dosage: 1–2 g/kg or 5–10 times the weight of the ingested poison, may be given q 4–6 hr.

Brands: 400 mg activated charcoal + 80 mg simethicone: Distenil tablet.
- If given along with milk, ice cream may reduce its effectiveness
- May cause vomiting, constipation, black stools, intestinal obstruction.

CHLORHEXIDINE

Uses: As antibacterial (sialadenitis, gingivitis prevention, mucositis, aphthous ulcer), hand and dental rinse, surgical scrub.

Dosage: Oral rinse—5–15 mL twice daily for 30 seconds to 1 minute. Cleanser: 5 mL per scrub or handwash. Dental gel: 1 inch gel brushed around the teeth and gums once or twice daily for 1 minute. Oral spray: 4–8 actuations/day.

Brands: 0.2% mouthwash; Clohex, Hexitrin, Rexidin. 4% solution; 0.2% lotion; Harifresh. 0.5% solution; Microgard. 5% gel; Oragine gel.
- Avoid eating for 2–3 hours after oral rinse. May cause skin and tongue irritation, staining of oral surface.

CHOLESTYRAMINE RESIN

Uses: Hypercholesterolemia, pruritus associated with elevated bile acids, diarrhea associated with excess fecal bile acids.

Dosage: PO—240 mg/kg/day divided q 8 hr (maximum: 8 g/day).

Brands: 4 g sachet; Questran.
- Avoid in biliary obstruction or atresia. For long-term therapy, multivitamin, iron and folic acid is recommended in addition. May cause constipation, malabsorption of fat-soluble vitamins, hyperchloremic acidosis. Avoid oral intake of other medications 2 hours before or after administration of resin.

CINNARIZINE

Uses: Motion sickness, vestibular disorders.

Dosage: Vestibular disorders: PO—5–12 years: 15 mg thrice daily. 12–18 years: 30 mg thrice daily. Motion sickness: PO—5–12 years: 15 mg, 2 hours before travel then 7.5 mg 8 hourly during travel if necessary. 12–18 years: 30 mg 2 hours before travel.

Brands: 25,75 mg tablet; Cintigo, Stugron.

COLOSTRUM

Uses: As immune modulator to provide antibodies.

Dosage: PO—44 mg/kg/day in divided doses.

Brands: 90 g pack; Pedimune powder.

- It is a pre-milk fluid produced in the first 48 hours after giving birth.

CYCLOPHOSPHAMIDE

Use and dosage:
- SLE: IV—500–750 mg/m^2 per month.
- Juvenile rheumatoid arthritis (JRA)/vasculitis: IV–10 mg/kg once in 2 weeks.
- Nephrotic syndrome: PO—2–3 mg/kg/day for upto 12 weeks.
- Idiopathic thrombocytopenic purpura (ITP): PO—1–2 mg/kg/day.

Brands: 500 mg tablet; Endoxan. 200, 500, 1000 mg vial; Endoxan-N, Cycloxan.

CYCLOSPORIN

Use and dosage:
- Juvenile idiopathic arthritis, Collagen disease, Vasculitis: PO—1–2 mg/kg/dose 2 times daily can be increased gradually upto 3 mg/kg/dose twice daily.
- Organ transplant: PO—5–7 mg/kg/dose 2 times daily starting 12 hours before transplant and continued for 1–2 weeks postoperative.
- Bone marrow transplantation—6–7.5 mg/kg/dose 2 times daily starting on day prior to transplant.

- Psoriasis/atopic dermatitis: 1.25 mg/kg /dose 2 times daily; increase if no response after 2 weeks for dermatitis and 4 weeks for psoriasis till 2.5 mg/kg/dose 2 times daily.

Brands: 100 mg/5 mL solution; Imusporin. 50,100 mg capsule; Imusporin, Oanimun, Graftin. 100 mg/mL injection; Immusol, Zymmune.

DESMOPRESSIN

Uses: Nocturnal enuresis, diabetes insipidus.

Dosages:
- Nocturnal enuresis: Intranasal in >5 years—20 µg once daily every night; half dose in each nostril for 3 months. Subsequent doses are to be titrated (maximum: 40 µg once daily).
- Diabetes insipedus (established disease): Given once or twice daily
  Birth-1 month: 1.25–5 µg
  1 month–2 years: 2.5–5 µg
  2–12 years: 5–20 µg
  12–18 years: 10–20 µg
- Individual dose titration is required.

Brands: 0.1 mg tablet; Minirin, Adiuretin. 10 µg/spray; D-void, Minirin, Adiuretin.

DEXTROMETHORPHAN

Uses: Symptomatic relief in nonproductive cough.

Dosage:
- 2–6 years: 2.5–7.5 mg q 8 hr (maximum: 30 mg/day)
- 7–12 years: 5–10 mg q 8 hr (maximum: 60 mg/day)
- >12 years: 10–30 mg q 8 hr (maximum: 120 mg/day).

Brands: 10 mg tablet; 30 mg/5 mL syrup; Lastuss. 10 mg/5 mL syrup; Suppressa.
- May cause drowsiness, dizziness, nausea.

DOXAPRAM

Uses: Treatment of apnea of prematurity not responding to theophylline therapy.

Dosage: Initial dose of 2.5 mg/kg followed by continuous infusion of 1 mg/kg/h (maximum: 2.5 mg/kg/h).

Brands: 20 mg/mL injection; Caropram, Dopram.

- Contraindication is seizures, cerebral edema, respiratory problem. May cause hypertension (HT), tachycardia, central nervous system (CNS) stimulation.

FLUNARIZINE

Uses: Migraine prophylaxis.

Dosage: PO– once daily.
- 3–12 years: 5 mg and >12 years: 10 mg.

Brands: 5 and 10 mg tablet; Flunarin, Sibelium, Nariz.

- Increased appetite after some time may lead to weight gain.

GASTROGRAFIN

Uses: Meconium ileus, distal intestinal obstructive disease, cystic fibrosis, imaging of gastrointestinal (GI) tract.

Dosage: Oral/rectal: <2 years, 15–30 mL. 15–25 kg: 50 mL: >25 kg: 100 mL.

For oral use in infants and young children should be diluted with 3 times its volume in water or fruit juice. May be given in divided doses if not tolerated. For rectal use in <5 years dilute with 5 times its volume in water, in >5 years dilute with 4 times its volume in water.

- Gastrografin may cause the loss of large amount of fluid into intestine, so intravenous pre-hydration should be maintained in neonates and infants.

GLUCAGON

Uses: Hypoglycemia treatment in children with type-1 diabetes or congenital hyperinsulinism, beta-blocker overdose.

Dosage: IV, IM, SC
- Neonates, infants and children <20 kg: 0.02–0.03 mg/ kg or 0.5 mg
- Children >20 kg: 1 mg.

Brands: 1 mg/mL vial; Glucagon novo.

GLYCOPYRROLATE

Uses: Inhibition of salivation and excessive secretions of the respiratory tract, reversal of muscarinic effects of cholinergic agents.

Dosage:
- Control of secretions: PO—40–100 µg/kg/dose 3–4 times/day and IM, IV—4–10 µg/kg/dose q 3–4 hr
- Preoperative: IM—4–5 µg/kg 30–60 minutes before procedure
- Reversal of muscarinic effects: IV—0.2 mg for each 1 mg of neostigmine and 5 mg of pyridostigmine administered.

Brands: 0.2 mg/mL injection; Glyprolate, Pyrolate.
- Infants with Down's syndrome, spastic paralysis or brain damage may be hypersensitive to its effects.

GUAIFENESIN

Uses: Symptomatic treatment of cough (expectorant).

Dosage: PO
- <2 years: 12 mg/kg/day in divided doses
- 2–5 years: 50–100 mg/kg/day
- >6 years: 100–200 mg q 4 hr.

Brands: Axalin expectorant: guaifenesin 50 mg + Dextromethorphan 5 mg + CPM 2.5 mg + Ammonium chloride 60 mg/5 mL. Codicoff expectorant: guaifenesin: 100 mg + Dextromethorphan 10 mg/5 mL. Dilo- BM expectorant: Ambroxol 30 mg + Guaiphenesin 30 mg + Terbutaline 1.25 mg/5 mL.

Administer with large quantity of fluid to ensure proper action.

HYDROXYUREA (HYDROXYCARBAMIDE)

Use and dosage:
- Sickle cell disease: 10–20 mg/kg/day and doses titrared as tolerated. (maximum: 35 mg/kg/day)
- Malignant glioma, astrocytoma, medulloblastoma, primitive neuroectodermal tumors: 1,500–3,000 mg/m^2 as a single dose every 4–6 weeks, given in combination with other agents.
- Acute myelogenous leukemia: 50–75 mg/kg/day.

Brands: 500 mg tablet; Urdox, Cytodrox, Hondrea. 500 mg capsule; Myelostat.

INSULIN

Uses: Treatment of insulin-dependent diabetes mellitus, hyperkalemia, diabetic ketoacidosis.

Dosage: Only regular insulin can be given IV or IM–
- Neonates: Regular insulin 0.01–0.1 unit/kg/h continuous infusion or 0.1–0.2 unit/kg q 6–12 hr SC.
- Children: 0.5–1 unit/kg/day in divided doses SC, adjust dose as per blood glucose level.
- Diabetic ketoacidosis: IV–loading dose of 0.1 unit/kg followed by maintenance continuous infusion of 0.1 unit/kg/h, adjust as per blood glucose level.
- Hyperkalemia (treat with IV calcium and sodium bicarbonate before giving insulin): Add 1 unit of regular insulin in 5g of dextrose solution, infuse at a rate of 0.5–1 g/kg over 30 minutes followed by 0.1unit/kg SC or IV.

Brands: 40 unit/mL (neutral) injection; Actrapid. 40 and 100 unit/mL (isophane) injection; Human Insulatard. 30% soluble + 70% isophane insulin 40 unit/mL injection; Huminsulin 30:70, Humstard 30:70. 50% soluble + 50% isophane insulin 40 and 100 unit/mL injection; Huminsulin 50:50.
- May cause hypoglycemia leading to palpitation, pallor, fatigue, confusion, nausea, numbness of mouth, tremor and hypokalemia; do not change brand once the blood glucose level is regulated
- Flush the tubing with 25 mL of insulin solution before beginning the infusion to reduce insulin loss due to adsorption.

INTRALIPID

Uses: Total parenteral nutrition to provide essential fatty acids.

Dosage: Dosage and infusion rates are determined by the ability to eliminate intralipid. 1 g triglycerides corresponds to 10 mL intralipid 10% or 5 mL intralipid 20%.

- Premature and low birth weight neonates: Initially 0.5–1g/kg/day followed by a successive increase by 0.5–1g/kg/day, only with close monitoring of serum triglycerides concentration.
- Neonates and infants: 0.5–4 g/kg/day. Rate of infusion should not exceed 0.17g triglycerides/kg/24 hr.

Brands: 10% Intralipid in 500 mL, 20% Intralipid in 250, 500 mL.

KETAMINE

Uses: Anesthesia for short procedure.

Dosage: Give ½ hour before procedure. IM—3–7 mg/kg. IV—0.5–2 mg/kg. Continuous infusion; 5–20 µg/kg/min.

Brands: 10 and 50 mg/mL injection; Ketalar, Ketam, Ketmin.
- Contraindicated in raised ICT, HT, CHF, psychotic disorders. Used in combination with anticholinergic agents to decrease salivation.

LOPERAMIDE

Uses: Short-term use for symptomatic relief in noninfective acute and chronic diarrhea, short bowel syndrome.

Dosage: PO; 2–5 years: 1 mg tds. 6–8 years: 2 mg bd. 8–12 years: 2 mg tds.

Brands: 2 mg tablet; Andial, Imodium, Ridol. 1 mg/5 mL syrup; Andial.
- May cause toxic megacolon and paralytic ileus.

METHOTREXATE

Uses and dosage:
- Juvenile idiopathic arthritis, juvenile dermatomyositis, vasculitis, uveitis, SLE, sarcoidosis: PO—SC/IM–child 1–18 years: 10–15 mg/m^2 once weekly.
- For all malignant conditions: Use doses prescribed in respective protocols.

Brands: 2.5 mg tablet; Alltrex, Methotrexate, Neotrexate. 15 mg/3 mL, 50 mg/2 mL injection; Alltrex.

MUPIROCIN

Uses: Impetigo, folliculitis, furunculosis, minor wounds, burns caused by *S. aureus* and *S. pyogenes*. Used intranasal to eradicate *S. aureus* carriers.

Dosage: Apply cream or ointment 2–3 times/day for 5–14 days.

Brands: 2% cream; Bactroban, Mupinova, 2% ointment; Bactroban, Mupirax, T-Bact.

OLANZAPINE

Uses: Schizophrenia, mania.

Dosage: PO—12–18 years: 5–20 mg once daily.

Brands: 5, 7.5, 10 mg tablet; Manza, Oliza, Opin.

ORAL REHYDRATION SOLUTION

Uses: Dehydration, acute diarrhea.

Dosage: Fluid and electrolyte loss in diarrhea: 1 month–1 year: 1–2 times usual feed volume. 1–12 years: 200 mL after every loose stool. 12–18 years: 200–400 mL after every loose stool.

Brands: 5.7, 28.5 g sachet; Electrobion

PANCREATIN

Uses: Pancreatic insufficiency.

Dosage: Dose varies widely and should be tailored to each individual according to symptoms, stool type, and abdominal findings. Dose varies from 5,000 to 10,000 units. Swallow tablet whole. Take with meal or snack.

Brands: Pancreatin 175 mg + Simethicone 50 mg + Charcoal 50 mg; Medizyme tablet. Pancreatin 192 mg + Bile constituents 25 mg + Dimethicon 40 mg; B-zyme tablet.

- Inadequate dosing may lead to steatorrhea and overdoses to impaction.

PANCURONIUM BROMIDE

Uses: Neuromuscular blockade, ventilation, anesthesia, surgical procedure.

Dosage:
- Newborn: IV–loading dose of 0.1 mg/kg followed by maintenance dose of 0.05 mg/kg/dose 4–6 times daily as needed.
- Children: IV—0.06–0.1 mg initially followed by 0.01–0.02 mg/kg as required.

Brands: 2 mg/mL injection; Pavulon. 4 mg/mL injection; Neocuron.
- Overdose is reversed by atropine (20 µg/kg) followed by IV neostigmine (80 µg/kg).

PHOLCODINE

Uses: Cough—dry and painfull.

Dasages: PO—given 3–4 times per day:
- 1 month–6 years: 2 mg/dose. 6–12 years: 2.5 mg/dose. 12–18 years: 5–10 mg/dose.

Brands: 1.5 mg/5 mL Pholcodine + 1.5 mg/5 mL Promethazine syrup; CRM, Tedykoff-LX.

PIRACETAM

Uses: Adjunct therapy in cerebral vascular accidents and cerebral insufficiencies; mental retardation; enhance memory and learning.

Dosage: PO—50 mg/kg/day in 3 divided doses (maximum: 400 mg/dose). Learning difficulties: 3 g/day in 3 divided doses for 1 school year.

Brands: 500 mg/5 mL syrup; 400 and 800 mg tablet; Ceretam, Nootropil, Sumocetam.
- May cause epigastric distress, CNS stimulation, excitement, sleep disturbance.

PROPOFOL

Uses: Induction and maintenance of general anesthesia, sedation, hypnotic.

Dosage: IV
- Induction of anesthesia: 1.5–2.5 mg/kg
- Maintenance of anesthesia: 9–15 mg/kg/hr
- Sedation: 1.5–3 mg/kg/dose over 1–2 minutes. Continuous sedation (mechanical ventilation): 5.5 mg/kg for 30 minutes and can be increased gradually upto 12.5 mg/kg/hr.

Brands: 1 and 2% vial for injection; Propovan. 10 mg/mL injection; Celofol, Rapifol.
- If required should be diluted in 5% glucose only; discard any left over after 6 hours
- Avoid abrupt discontinuation of infusion.

PROSTAGLANDIN E1

Uses: To maintain patency of ductus in ductus-dependent congenital heart diseases.

Dosage:
- Continuous infusion: 0.05–0.1µg/kg/min in a large vein or umbilical artery catheter at the level of ductus arteriosus.
- Maintenance dose is 0.01µg/kg/min, after the ductus is opened.

Brands: 500 µg/mL injection; Alpostin, Prostin VR.

RACECADOTRIL

Uses: Symptomatic relief in diarrhea.

Dosage: PO—1.5 mg/kg 3times/day.

Brands: 100 mg capsule; 10 and 30 mg sachet; Racedot, Raceloc, Zedott.

SACCHAROMYCES BOULARDII

Uses: Acute infectious/antibiotic-induced diarrhea, irritable bowel syndrome, diarrhea in tube fed infants.

Dosage: PO—250–500 mg/day for 5–7 days in single or two divided doses.

Brands: Each lyophilized sachet contain 282.5 mg of *S. boulardii* equivalent to 250 mg of yeast; Solib, Stibs.
- Generally safe in normal, previously healthy infants and children, but should be avoided in very ill and immune-compromised individuals.

SELENIUM SULFIDE

Uses: Seborrheic dermatitis, tinea versicolor, dandruff.

Dosage: Topical in >2 years

- Tinea versicolor: Apply and leave for 30 minutes and then rinse
- Dandruff, seborrhea: Apply twice weekly for 2 weeks then once weekly for 4 weeks. Apply and leave for 5–10 minutes and then rise.

Brands: 2.5% liquid; Selsun, Seldan.

- Avoid contact with eyes and inflamed skin.

SILDENAFIL

Uses: Persistant pulmonary hypertension of the newborn, vasodilator, idiopathic pulmonary artery HT (class-1), Pulmonary HT secondary to connective tissue disorders (class-1).

Dosage: PO:
- Neonate : 0.3–1 mg/kg/dose q 8–12 hr.
- Infant and children: 0.25–0.5 mg/kg/dose q 8 hr.

Brands: 25, 50 mg tablet; Alsigra, Progra, Silagra, Jvan.

- Use with caution in sepsis, hepatic, and renal problems.

SILYMARIN

Uses: Infective hepatitis, chronic active hepatitis, toxic metabolic hepatic damage, supportive treatment in cirrhosis, carbon tetrachloride poisoning, mushroom poisoning.

Dosages: PO—70–140 mg bd/tds.

Brands: 35 mg/5 mL suspension; 140 mg tablet; Limarin, Silybon.

SIMETHICONE (ACTIVATED DIMETHICONE)

Uses: Relieves flatulence, functional gastric bloating, postoperative gas pain.

Dosage: PO—<2 years: 20 mg/dose q 4–6 hr. 2–12 years: 40 mg/dose q 6 hr. >12 years: 40–120 mg q 6 hr.

Brands: 40 mg/mL drops; Dimol, Siflat. 40 mg tablet; Dimol. Simethicone 80 mg + Charcoal 400 mg tablet; Gasnil.

SUCROSE SOLUTION

Uses: As analgesic in preterm and term infants.

Dosage: PO
- Preterm: <28 weeks; 0.2 mL. 28–32 weeks; 0.2–2 mL. >32 weeks; 2 mL
- Term: 1.5–2 mL
  - Give the required dose over 1–2 minutes; dose may be repeated once if required. Analgesic effect may last for up to 8 minutes; wait for 2 minutes before starting procedure.

SURFACTANT

Uses: Prophylaxis and treatment of respiratory distress syndrome (RDS) in premature neonates.

Dosage:
- Survanta: Prophylactic therapy– 4 mL/kg/dose intratracheally as soon as possible; up to 4 doses can be given at 6 hours interval during the first 48 hours of life. Rescue therapy: 4 mL/kg/dose intratracheally, immediately following the diagnosis of RDS. May repeat 4 dose as needed at 6 hours interval.
- Curosurf: Intratracheal—1.25 mL/kg over 4 minutes; repeat after 12 hours if required. If birth weight is <1,250 g, give first dose within 15 minutes of birth.
- Exosurf: Intratracheal– 67.5 mg/kg or 5 mL/kg. Second and third dose if required can be given after 12 and 24 hours later.

Brands: Suspension for inhalation; 25 mg/mL; Survanta. 80 mg/ml vial; Curosurf. 33.75 mg/2.5 mL vial; Exosurf.

Method of administration: Suction infant prior to administration. Give via a 5F feeding tube. Each dose is divided into four 1 mL/kg aliquots; administer 1 mL/kg in each of four different positions over 2–3 s.
- May cause bradycardia, pallor, hypotension, apnea, pulmonary air leak, etc.

TACROLIMUS

Uses: As immunosuppressant in organ transplant, topically for severe atopic dermatitis.

Dosage:
- Children: PO—0.2 mg/kg q 12 hr
- Topical: Apply 0.02% ointment locally twice.

Brands: 1 and 5 mg tablet; Crolium. 0.5, 1, and 5 mg capsule; Tacromus. 0.02% ointment; Tacroderm, Tacrovate.

TINOCARDIA

Promote leukocytosis with prominant effect on neutrophils and also enhances phagocytic capacity.

Uses: Adjuvant in chronic illness (recurrent tonsilitis, chronic otitis media, tuberculosis, bronchial asthma, etc.).

Dosage: PO—100 mg thrice daily in children >3 years.

Brands: 100 and 500 mg tablet; 200 mg/5 mL syrup; Immumod.

URSODEOXYCHOLIC ACID

Uses: Prevention and dissolution of small cholesterol gallstones, cholestatic conditions, such as primary biliary cirrhosis, severe hepatic dysfuntion.

Dosage: PO—10–15 mg/kg/day in 1–2 divided doses.

Brands: 150 and 300 mg tablet; Udihep, Udiliv, Urso. 75 mg tablet; Actibile.
- Contraindication: Calcified cholesterol stones, gallstones >15 mm, hepatic impairment, biliary obstruction.

Appendices

APPENDIX 1: TABLES

Table 1: Equipment for resuscitation in various age group.

Equipment	Premature	New-born	6 months	1–2 years	5 years	8–10 years
Chest tubes	10–14 F	12–18 F	14–20 F	14–24 F	20–32 F	28–38 F
NG tubes	5 feeding	5–8 feeding	8 F	10 F	10–12 F	14–18 F
Foley's	5 feeding	5–8 feeding	8 F	10 F	10–12 F	12 F
O_2 masks	Newborn	Newborn	Pediatric	Pediatric	Pediatric	Adult
ET tubes	2.5–3.0	3–3.5	3.5–4.5	4.0–4.5	5.0–5.5	5.5–6.5
Arm boards	6 inch	6 inch	6–8 inch	8 inch	8–15 inch	15 inch
BP cuff	Newborn	Newborn	Infant or child	Child	Child	Child or adult
Laryngo-scope blade	0	1	1	1	2	Adult

(NG: nasogastric; NB: newborn; ET: endotracheal; BP: blood pressure)

Table 2: Fasting guidelines for sedation or anesthesia.

Food	Hours of fasting required
Clear liquids	2
Breast milk	2–4
Formula or light meal (no fat)	6
Full meal	8

Table 3: Sedation techniques suggested for children.

Procedure	Sedation and analgesia technique

Lumbar puncture	• Local anesthesia with minimal/moderate sedation:
	  – Local anesthetics: Lidocaine/EMLA cream
	  – Minimal/moderate sedation: Midazolam or sometimes
	• Deep sedation: Fentanyl/Midazolam or Ketamine

Painful procedures: Biopsy of liver/kidney, bone marrow aspiration, fracture reduction, drainage of abscess, burn debridement	Deep sedation combined with local anesthesia: As above
Laceration repair	Local anesthesia with minimal/moderate/deep sedation: As above
Intravenous catheter placement	Local anesthesia and sometimes minimal/moderate sedation: As above

Table 4: Drip calculations.

Drug	Dose	Calculation	Rate and dose
Dobutamine	5–20 µg/kg/min	6 × body weight (kg) is the milligram added to make 100 mL	1 mL/h = 1 µg/kg/min
Dopamine	2–20 µg/kg/min	6 × body weight (kg) is the milligram added to make 100 mL	1 mL/h = 1 µg/kg/min
Epinephrine	0.1–1 µg/kg/min	0.6 × body weight (kg) is the milligram added to make 100 mL	1 mL/h = 0.1 µg/kg/min
Isoproterenol	0.1–1 µg/kg/min	0.6 × body weight (kg) is the milligram added to make 100 mL	1 mL/h = 0.1 µg/kg/min
Lidocaine	20–50 µg/kg/min	120 mg in 100 mL of D5%	1 mL/kg/h = 20 µg/kg/min

- Patients ≤40 kg and those requiring fluid restriction may need more concentrated solutions in order to deliver less fluid per hour. In those cases or as an alternative to the listed calculations above, use the following equation:

$$\text{Rate (mL/h)} = \frac{\text{Dose } (\mu g/kg/min) \times \text{weight (kg)} \times 60 \text{ min/h}}{\text{Concentration } (\mu g/mL)}$$

Table 5: Treatment for drug extravasation.

Medication extravasated	Cold/warm pack	Treatment
Ischemic inducer		
Dobutamine, dopamine, epinephrine, norepinephrine, phenyleprine, vasopressin	None	Phentolamine: Mix 5 mg with 9 mL of normal saline (NS). Inject a small amount of this solution into extravasated area. Blanching should reverse immediately. Monitor site, if blanching recur, additional injections of phentolamine may be needed
Miscellaneous agents		
Aminophylline, calcium salts, dextrose, mannitol, phenytoin, contrast media, sodium bicarbonate, sodium chloride, tetracycline	Cold	Hyaluronidase: Add 1 mL NS to 150 units to make 15 units/mL. Administer 0.2 mL SC or intradermally into the extravasated site

Table 6: Estimation of total body surface area of burn involvement (% by site and age).

Site	0–1 years	1–4 years	5–9 years	10–14 years	15 years	Adult
Head	9.5	8.5	6.5	5.5	4.5	3.5
Neck	0.5	0.5	0.5	0.5	0.5	0.5
Trunk	13	13	13	13	13	13
Upper arm	2	2	2	2	2	2
Forearm	1.5	1.5	1.5	1.5	1.5	1.5
Hand	1.5	1.5	1.5	1.5	1.5	1.5
Perineum	1	1	1	1	1	1
Buttock	2.5	2.5	2.5	2.5	2.5	2.5
Thigh	2.75	3.25	4	4.25	4.5	4.75
Leg	2.5	2.5	2.75	3.00	3.25	3.5
Foot	1.75	1.75	1.75	1.75	1.75	1.75

Note:
- The total body surface area of burn involvement is determined by the sum of the percentages of each site.
- Applicable to second and third degree burns.
- Percentage for each site is only for a single extremity with anterior or posterior involvement. Percentage should be doubled if both anterior and posterior involvement of a single extremity.

PARKLAND FLUID REPLACEMENT FORMULA

A guideline for replacement of deficits and ongoing losses (note: For infants, maintenance fluids may need to be added to this). Administer 4 mL/kg/percentage burn of Ringer's lactate (glucose may be added but beware of stress hyperglycemia) over the first 24 hours; half of this total is given over the first 8 hours calculated from the time of injury; the remaining half is given over the next 16 hours. The second 24 hours fluid requirements average 50–75% of first day's requirements. Concentrations and rates best determined by monitoring weight, serum electrolytes, urine output, nasogastric (NG) losses, etc.

Colloid may be added after 18–24 hours (1 g/kg/day of albumin) to maintain serum albumin >2 g/100 mL.

Potassium is generally with held for the first 48 hours due to the large amount of potassium that is released from damaged tissues. To manage serum electrolytes, monitor urine electrolytes twice weekly and replace calculated urine losses.

Table 7: Average weight and surface area.

Age	Average weight (kg)*	Approximate surface area (m²)
Weeks gestation		
26	0.9–1	0.1
30	1.3–1.5	0.12
32	1.6–2	0.15
38	2.9–3	0.2
40 (term infant at birth)	3.1–4	0.25
Months		
3	5	0.29
6	7	0.38
9	8	0.42
Years		
1	10	0.49
2	12	0.55
3	15	0.64
4	17	0.74
5	18	0.76
6	20	0.82
7	23	0.90
8	25	0.95
9	28	1.06

Contd...

Contd...

10	33	1.18
11	35	1.23
12	40	1.34
Adult	70	1.73

*Weights from age 3 months and over are rounded off to the nearest kilogram.

Table 8: Calculation of surface area from weight.

Weight range	Surface area
1–5 kg	(0.05 × weight) + 0.05
6–10 kg	(0.04 × weight) + 0.10
11–20 kg	(0.04 × weight) + 0.20
21–40 kg	(0.02 × weight) + 0.40

Table 9: Quick reference chart for Intravenous medication.

Drug	Maximum concentration	Maximum rate
Acyclovir	10 mg/mL	Give over 1 hour
Adenosine	3 mg/mL	Give over 1–2 seconds
Amikacin	10 mg/mL	Give over 30 minutes
Aminophylline	25 mg/mL	25 mg/minutes
Amphotericin B	0.1 mg/mL	Give over 2–6 hours
Ampicillin	100 mg/mL	10 mg/kg/min
Atropine	1 mg/mL	Give over 1 minutes
Calcium gluconate	100 mg/mL	100 mg/min
Cefazolin	20 mg/mL	Give over 10–60 minutes
Cefepime	160 mg/mL	Give over 30 minutes
Cefotaxime	60 mg/mL	Give over 10–30 minutes
Ceftazidime	40 mg/mL	Give over 10–30 minutes
Ceftriaxone	40 mg/mL	Give over 10–30 minutes

Contd...

Contd...

Cefuroxime	30 mg/mL	Give over 15–60 minutes
Dexamethasone	10 mg/mL	Doses <10 mg give over 1–4 minutes Doses >10 mg give over 10–20 minutes
Diazepam	5 mg/mL	2 mg/min
Digoxin	100 µg/mL	Give over 5 minutes
Fosphenytoin	25 mg/mL	3 mg/kg/min
Gentamicin	40 mg/mL	Give over 30 minutes
Hydrocortisone	5 mg/mL	Give over 20–30 minutes
Ketamine	2 mg/mL	0.5 mg/kg/min
Lorazepam	4 mg/mL	0.05 mg/kg over 2–5 minutes
Meropenem	50 mg/mL	Give over 15–30 minutes
Methylprednisolone	2.5 mg/mL	Give over 20–60 minutes
Metoclopramide	5 mg/mL	Give over 1–2 minutes
Metronidazole	8 mg/mL	Give over 1 hour
Midazolam	5 mg/mL	Give over 20–30 seconds (5 minutes in neonates)
Ondansetron	2 mg/mL	Give over 2–15 minutes
Phenobarbital	130 mg/mL	2 mg/kg/min
Phenytoin	50 mg/mL	3 mg/kg/min
Piperacillin	20 mg/mL	Give over 20–30 minutes
Ranitidine	2.5 mg/mL	10 mg/min
Vancomycin	5 mg/mL	Give over 60 minutes

In infants and children risk of fluid overload is always a consideration, when giving IV medications. Following table provides maximum concentrations and the maximum rate at which the medications can be given.

Table 10: Identifying the acid bare disorder.

Primary disorder	Initial change	Compensatory change
Metabolic acidosis	↓ HCO_3^-	↓ $PaCO_2$
Metabolic alkalosis	↑ HCO_3^-	↑ $PaCO_2$
Respiratory acidosis	↑ $PaCO_2$	↑ HCO_3^-
Respiratory alkalosis	↓ $PaCO_2$	↓ HCO_3^-

Table 11: Equivalent values of salts.

1g NaCl	=	18 mEq Na, Cl
1g $NaHCO_3$	=	12 mEq Na, HCO_3
1g KCl	=	14 mEq K, Cl
1g $CaCl_2$	=	20 mEq Ca
1g calcium gluconate	=	4.5 mEq Ca
1g $MgSO_4$	=	8.3 mEq Mg
1 mEq Na	=	59 mg NaCl
1 mEq Na	=	84 mg $NaHCO_3$
1 mEq Na	=	112 Na Lactate
1 mEq K	=	74.5 mg KCl
1 mEq Ca	=	55 mg $CaCl_2$
1 mEq Ca	=	224 mg Ca gluconate
1 mEq Mg	=	120 mg $MgSO_4$

Table 12: Difference between arterial blood gases (ABG) and venous blood gases (VBG).

	Arterial	*Venous*
pH	7.35–7.45	0.04 units less
PaO_2	95 mm Hg	40 mm Hg
$PaCO_2$	35–45 mm Hg	5–7 mm Hg more
SaO_2	97%	75%

Table 13: Parenteral nutrition initation and maintenance guidelines.

Substrate	*Initiation*	*Advancement*	*Goals*
Dextrose	10%	2–5% /day	25%
Amino acid	1 g/kg/day	0.5–1 g/kg/day	2–3 g/kg/day
20% lipids	1 g/kg/day	0.5–1 g/kg/day	2–3 g/kg/day

Table 14: Electrolyte requirement during parenteral nutrition.

Sodium	2–4 mEq/kg/day
Potassium	2–3 mEq/kg/day
Magnesium	0.25–0.5 mEg/kg/day
Calcium	Neonate: 50–100 mg/kg/day Infant: 100–200 mg/kg/day Adolescent: 50–100 mg/kg/day
Phosphate	30–70 mg/kg/day

Table 15: Fraction of inspired oxygen (FiO_2) delivered by various devices.

	FiO_2 delivered	*Flow required*
Nasal cannula	24–50%	2–4 L
Face mask	40%	4–5 L
Venturi mask	40–60%	6–8 L
Nonrebreathing mask	80%	6–8 L
Under hood	95%	10 L

Table 16: Initial ventilator settings in neonates.

Disease	PIP	Peep	Ti	I:E ratio	RR	FiO$_2$
Moderate RDS	18–20	4–5	0.4	1:2	40–50	0.5
Severe RDS	23–25	5	0.4	1:2	40–50	0.9–1.0
Apnea of prematurity	12–14	3–4	0.4–0.5	1:2	30–40	0.21–0.3
MAS	16–20	2–3	0.4–0.5	1:3–4	30	0.9–1.0

(RDS: respiratory distress syndrome; MAS: meconium aspiration syndrome; PIP: peak inspiratory pressure; PEEP: positive end-expiratory pressure, I:E ratio: inspiratory:expiratory ratio; RR: respiratory rate)

Table 17: Rapid sequence intubation drugs.

Drug	Dose	Comments
First (adjuncts)		
Atropine	0.01–0.02 mg/kg Minimum: 0.1 mg Maximum: 1 mg	Prevents bradycardia and prevents oral secretions
Sedative-hypnotic (second line)		
Thiopental or	1–5 mg/kg	Contraindicated in asthmatics Decreases BP Avoid in hypotensive child
Ketamine or	1–4 mg/kg	May increase BP, ICP, HR and oral secretions, causes bronchodilatation
Midazolam or	0.05–0.1 mg/kg	May decrease BP, HR Respiratory depression
Fentanyl or	1–5 µg/kg	Fewest hemodynamic effects Chest wall rigidity
Etomidate	0.2–0.3 mg/kg	Does not cause hypotension or Increased ICP

Contd...

Contd...

Paralytic (third line)		
Rocuronium or	0.6–1.2 mg/kg	Onset—30 seconds, duration 30–60 minutes Minimal effect on hemodynamics Flush line before and after use
Vecuronium or	0.1–0.2 mg/kg	Onset :70–120 seconds, duration—30–90 minutes, minimal effect on BP/HR Reversal of effect with atropine or neostigmine within 30 minutes
Succinylcholine	1–2 mg/kg	Onset—30–60 seconds, duration—3–10 minutes, increases ICP, contraindicated in burns, massive trauma, neuromuscular disorder, malignant hyperthermia and pseudocholinesterase deficiency

(BP: blood pressure, ICP: intracranial pressure; HR: heart rate)

Table 18: Properties of common Intravenous fluids and its composition.

Solution	Na	Cl	K	Ca	Lactate	Kcal/L	mOsm
D5W	0	0	0	0	0	170	252
D10W	0	0	0	0	0	340	505
D50W	0	0	0	0	0	1700	2530
½ NS	77	77	0	0	0	0	154
NS	154	154	0	0	0	0	308
3% NaCl	513	513	0	0	0	0	1026
RL	130	109	4	3	28	0	273
20% mannitol	0	0	0	0	0	0	1098

(NS: normal saline)

Table 19: Average pulse, blood pressure (BP), body surface area (BSA).

Age	Weight (kg)	Surface area (m²)	Pulse 95% range	Mean BP 95% range
Term	3.5	0.23	95–145	40–60
3 months	6	0.31	110–175	45–75
6 months	7.5	0.38	110–175	50–90
1 year	10	0.47	105–170	50–100
3 years	14	0.61	82–140	50–100
7 years	22	0.86	70–120	60–90
10 years	30	1.10	60–110	60–90
12 years	38	1.30	60–100	65–95

APPENDIX 2: ADMINISTERING MEDICINES TO CHILDREN

Medication administration to a pediatric population is a very difficult job. One child may take the particular product and form of medicine easily, but the another child may not accept the same.

Nurses and residents should learn following points for administering medicines to children:

- In children oral route is preferred over parenteral. If not accepting one type of oral form try another form.
- Special equipments are available for administering oral medicines, e.g., measuring cups and spoons, oral syringes, oral droppers, cylindrical dosing spoons. Parents should be taught to use calibrated devices provided with product rather then using household utensils.
- In young children, it is better to give part of the dose at a time into the side of the cheek away from the bitter taste buds at the back of the tongue.
- Prefer liquid preparation in children <5 years of age and in >5 years of age give dispersible or chewable form of medicines.
- Maximum volume allowed in parenteral administration is subcutaneous = 0.5, intradermal = 0.01–1 mL, intramuscular = 0.5–1 mL, intravenous = use smallest recommended diluent for dilution.
- For IM prefer shorter (½–1 inch) and smaller (23–30 G) needles.
- Give IV via pediatric drip set with microdrip chamber.
- For ID route use 1 mL syringes caliberated in 0.01 mL units 26–27 G needles.
- For SC route use 1 mL syringes caliberated in 40 or 80 units and 25 G needles.
- Always compare the ordered dose with the recommended formulary dose based on a child's weight or BSA. Ordered dose is considered safe if it is less than or equal to the recommended formulary dose.

APPENDIX 3: GENERAL INSTRUCTIONS ON IMMUNIZATION

- Vaccination at birth means as early as possible or within 24–72 hours after birth or at least not later than 1 week after birth.
- Whenever multiple vaccination are to be given simultaneously, they should be given within 24 hours if simultaneous administration is not feasible due to some reasons.
- The recommended age in weeks/months/years means completed weeks/months/years.
- Any dose not administered at the recommended age should be administered at a subsequent visit, when indicated and possible.
- Equivalent component vaccine combination use is preferred over separate injections.
- When two or more live parenteral vaccines are not administered on the same day, they should be given at least 28 days apart. This does not apply to administration of live oral vaccines.
- There should be a gap of 4 weeks between administration of two in activated vaccines (this does not apply to rabies vaccination).
- Different vaccines should not be mixed in the same syringe.
- Patients should be observed for 15–20 minutes after vaccination in the clinic and hospital.
- If necessary two vaccines can be given in the same limb at a single visit.
- The distance separating two vaccines in the same limb should be minimum of 1 inch, so that local reaction do not overlap.
- The anterolateral aspect of the thigh is the preferred site for two simultaneous intramuscular injections.

APPENDIX 4: AGE-BASED FORMULA FOR SELECTING ENDOTRACHEAL TUBE SIZE (INTERNAL DIAMETER IN MILLIMETER)

$$\text{Uncuffed tube size (mm)} = \frac{\text{Age (years)}}{4} + 4$$

$$\text{Cuffed tube size (mm)} = \frac{\text{Age (years)}}{4} + 3$$

Index

Page numbers followed by *t* refer to table.

A

Abacavir 123
Acetaminophen 5
    toxicity 59
Acetazolamide 155
Acetylcysteine 59
Acetylsalicylic acid 1
Acid-base
    disorder 228*t*
    imbalance 163
Acne 36, 185
    drug 185
    vulgaris 47
Acrodermatitis enteropathica 173
Actinomyces 34
Acute gout 3
    arthritis 86
Acute iron
    intoxication 145
    poisoning 145
Acyclovir 137, 226
Adapalene 185
Adefovir 138
Adenine 138
Adenosine 17, 226
Adrenal hyperplasia, congenital 152
Adrenal insufficiency 152
Adrenocortical insufficiency 151
Adrenocorticotropin hormone 176
Albendazole 88
Albumin 178
Alfacalcidol 174
Allergy 93
    conjunctivitis 92, 95
    problem 153
    rhinitis 12, 92, 93, 95
Allopurinol 86
Alprazolam 206
Amantadine 138
Amebiasis 115
Amikacin 22, 128, 226
Amiloride 155, 156
Aminocaproic acid 159
Aminoglycosides 21
    nephrotoxicity 22
Aminophylline 11, 226
Amiodarone 17
Amitriptyline 56
Amlodipine 97
Amniocentesis 165
Amoxicillin 37, 38
Amphotericin B 80, 115, 226
Ampicillin 38, 39, 226
Amprenavir 124
Amrinone 143
Amyl nitrite 60
Analgesic 1
Anaphylactic reaction 179, 187
Anaphylaxis 133
Ankylosing spondylitis 2, 3
Anthelmintics 88

Antiarrhythmics 17
Antiasthmatics 11
Antibiotics 21
Anticoagulants 54
Antidepressant 56, 58
Antidiphtheric serum 134
Antidotes 59, 64
Antiemetic 65
    therapy 73
Antiepileptics 69
Antifungal agent 80
Antigout agents 86
Antihemophilic factor 159
Antihistamines 92
Antihypertensives 97
Antileprotics 105
Antimalarials, drugs for 112
Antimicrobials, miscellaneous 47
Antimyasthenics 113
Antiprotozoals 115
Antipsychotics 118
Antiretrovirals 122
Antisecretory 135
Antisnake venom 133
Antispasmodics drugs 131
Antithyroid agent 190
Antitoxins 133
Antitubercular drugs 126
Antiulcers 135
Antivirals 137
Anxiety 73
Anxiolytics 118
Aripiprazole 56
Arrhythmia 101
    etiology of 17
Arteether 108
Artemether 108
Arterial blood gases 229*t*
Artesunate 108
Arthritis 5
    juvenile chronic 151
Ascariasis 89

Ascorbic acid 203
Aspergilosis 81
Astemizole 92
Asthma 13, 151, 153, 194
    bronchodilator in 15
    bronchospasm in 14
    chronic 13
    long-term control of 11, 12
    therapy of 12
    treatment of 13, 14, 16
Atenolol 97
Atomoxetin 118, 206
Atopic dermatitis 151
Atorvastatin 206
Atrial fibrillation 19
Atrial tachyarrhythmias 19
Atropine 59, 226
    sulfate 18
    toxicity 63
Attack, acute 110
Attention deficit hyperactivity
        syndrome 119
Auranofin 2
Autism spectrum disorder 56
Azatadine 92
Azathioprine 206
Azelaic acid 185
Azelastine 92
Azithromycin 35
Aztreonam 47

B

Bacillus Calmette-Guérin 192
Baclofen 63
Bacterial infection, acute 166
Bacterial meningitis 151
Bacteroids 34
Bambuterol 11
Beclomethasone 12
Bedaquiline 128
Benzocaine 9

Benzodiazepine toxicity 62
Benzoyl peroxide 185
Benztropine 60
Benzyl benzoate 180
Beparine 55
Betamethasone 150
Biotin 200
Biotinidase deficiency, primary 200
Bipolar disorders 58
Bisacodyl 169
Bleeding
    disorders, history of 1
    drugs for controlling 159
Blood cells, kind of 147
Botulinum A toxin 182
Bronchial asthma 12, 95
    treatment of 11
Bronchopulmonary dysplasia 141, 194
Bronchospasm 187
Budesonide 12
Bumetanide 155, 156
Bupropion 57
Burns, degree of 51

C

Caffeine citrate 207
Calamine lotion 186, 207
Calcium
    deficiency 161
    folinate 64
    gluconate 64, 161, 226
    phosphate 161, 174
    polystyrene sulfonate 207
Camplylobacter 27
Candida 80
Candidal oral thrush 82
Candidiasis 81
Capreomycin 128
Captopril 98
Carbamazepine 69

Carbapenem 25
Carbenicillin 39
Carbimazole 190
Carbon monoxide poisoning 62
Cardiac arrest 161, 163, 187
Cardiac failure 158
Cardiac shocks 143
Cardiovascular disease 1
Carnitine 174
    deficiency, treatment of 174
Carvedilol 98
Caspofungin 81
Cefaclor 28
Cefadroxil 27
Cefazolin 27, 226
Cefdinir 31
Cefditoren pivoxil 28
Cefepime 31, 226
Cefixime 32
Cefoperazone 30
Cefotaxime 29, 226
Cefpirome 33
Cefpodoxime 32
Cefprozil 32
Ceftazidime 31, 226
Ceftibuten 33
Ceftizoxime 33
Ceftriaxone 29, 226
Cefuroxime 28, 227
Celecoxib 2
Central nervous system 115, 162
Cephalexin 33
Cephalosporins 27
Cerebral edema 151, 178
Cerebral malaria 108
Cerebral spasticity, treatment of 182
Cetirizine 93
Chancroid 36
Charcoal 60, 208
Chelating agents 145
Chickenpox vaccine 198
Chlamydia 45, 46

Chloramphenicol 48
Chlordiazepoxide 118
Chlorhexidine 208
Chloroquine 109, 115
    resistant falciparum malaria 108, 111
Chlorothiazide 155
Chlorpheniramine maleate 93
Chlorpromazine 60, 68, 118
Chlorthalidone 156
Chlorzoxazone 183
Cholecalciferol 204
Cholera 36
Cholestyramine resin 208
Chronic iron 145
Ciclesonide 12
Cidofovir 138
Cimetidine 164
Cinnarizine 209
Ciprofloxacin 43
Clarithromycin 35, 105, 129
Clavulanic acid 38, 43
Clemastine fumarate 93
Clindamycin 34, 111, 112
Clobazam 70
Clobetasone 151, 186
Clofazimine 105, 129
Clonazepam 70
Clonidine 98, 119
Clostridium difficile 27, 52
Clotrimazole 81
Cloxacillin 39
Codeine 6
Colchicine 86
Colistimethate sodium 48
Colistin sulfate 48
Collagen diseases 153
Colony-stimulating factors 147
Colostrum 209
Coma 170
Congestive heart failure 199
Conjunctivitis 45, 92
Constipation 170
Control blood pressure 97
Corneal ulcers 45
Corticosteroids 150
Cortisone 151
Corynebacterium 49
Cough, nonproductive 6
Crotamiton 180
Crystalline penicillin 40
Cyanide kit 60
Cyanocobalamin 200
Cyanotic spells 101
Cyclophosphamide 209
Cycloserine 126, 129, 201
Cyclosporin 209
Cyproheptadine hydrochloride 93
Cystic fibrosis 3

D

Dantrolene 183
Dapsone 105, 106
Daptomycin 48
Deferasirox 145
Deferiprone 60, 145
Deflazacort 151
Delamanid 129
Delisprin tablet 1
Delusions 121
Demeclocycline 46
Dental caries, prevention of 172
Dental pain 5
Depression 56-58
Desferrioxamine 60, 145
Desloratadine 94
Desmopressin 176, 210
Dexamethasone 68, 151, 227
Dextran 179
Dextromethorphan 210
Dextrose 162
Dhatura poisoning 63
Diabetes insipidus 144, 176

Diazepam 71, 227
Diazoxide 99
Diclofenac sodium 2
Dicyclomine 131
Didanosine 123
Diethylcarbamazine 89
Digitalis glycoside toxicity 61
Digoxin 143, 227
    immune fab 61
Diloxanide furoate 115
Diltiazem 99
Dimenhydrinate 65
Dimercaprol 61, 146
Dimercaptosuccinic acid 61
Dimethicone, activated 218
Diphenhydramine 61, 94
Diphtheria 36, 192
    and tetanus 192
        prophylaxis 192
    antitoxin 134
Disopyramide 19
Diuretics 155
Dobutamine 102, 187, 222, 223
Domperidone 65
Dopamine 102, 188, 222, 223
Dosage 18
Down's syndrome 194
Doxapram 210
Doxepin 57
Doxophylline 13
Doxycycline 46, 111, 112
D-penicillamine 61, 146
Drip calculations 222*t*
Drotaverine 131
Drug extravasation, treatment for 223*t*
Duodenal ulcer 136
Dystonic reaction, acute 60

E

Ear infection 45
Ebastine 94

Ecosprin tablet 1
Edmonston-Zagreb strain vaccine 195
Edrophonium 64, 113
Efavirenz 124
Enalapril 99
Endogenous depression 56
Endorphins 6
Enoxaparin 54
Enterobacter 22, 23
Enterobiasis 89
Enterobius 88
Enuresis 57
Eosinophilia 34
Ephedrine 188
Epilepsy, partial 75
Epinephrine 11, 102, 187, 222, 223
Ertapenem 26
Erythromycin 36
Erythropoietin 147
Esomeprazole 135
Ethacrynic acid 156
Ethambutol 127
Ethamsylate 159
Ethanol 62
Ethionamide 127
Ethosuximide 71
Ethylene glycol 62
Etodolac 2
Etoricoxib 3
Eukephlins 6
Excessive bleeding, treatment of 159
Extrapulmonary tuberculosis 126
Eye infection 45, 46

F

Factor IX 160
Falciparum malaria 107

Famciclovir 138
Famotidine 164
Fat emulsion 175
Febrile neutropenia
 high-risk of 149
 prevention of 147
Fentanyl 7
Fexofenadine 94
Filariasis 89
Filgrastim 147
Flouroquinolones 105
Fluconazole 81
Flucytosine 82
Fludrocortisone 152
Flumazenil 62
Flunarizine 211
Fluoride 172
Fluoxetine 57
Fluticasone 13
Folic acid 201
Formoterol 13
Foscarnet 139
Fosfomycin 49
Fosphenytoin 72, 227
Framycetin 22
Furazolidone 49
Furosemide 156
Fusidic acid 49
Fusobacterium 34

G

Gabapentin 72
Gamma benzene hexachloride 181
Ganciclovir 139
Gas gangrene antitoxin 134
Gastric ulcer 136
Gastroesophageal reflux disease 135
Gastrografin 211
Gastrointestinal bleeding 1
Gatifloxacin 44
Gelatin 179

Gentamicin 227
Gentian violet 82
Giardia 49
Giardiasis 88, 115
Glucagon 62, 211
Glucose-6-phosphate
 dehydrogenase 106
Glycopyrrolate 212
Gonadotropin releasing hormone 177
Gouty arthritis
 chronic 86
 prevention of 87
Gram-negative
 bacilli 22, 24
 organisms 31
Gram-positive
 organisms 31
 Staphylococcus 23
Granisetron 66
Granulocyte-macrophage colony-
 stimulating factor 148
Griseofulvin 82
Guaifenesin 212
Guillain-Barre syndrome 166

H

H_2 antagonists 164
Haemophilus 30
 influenzae 192, 193
Hallucination 121
Haloperidol 119
Hamycin 82
Hansen disease 105
Heart disease
 chronic 194
 congenital 141
 cyanotic congenital 194
Heart failure 144
Helminth infections 115
Hemolytic anemia 145

Hemorrhage, transplacental 165
Hemorrhagic disease 205
Hemorrhoids 9
Heparin 54, 55
Hepatic encephalopathy 51, 170
Hepatitis
  A 193
  B 193
    prophylaxis 193
Herpes simplex conjunctivitis 142
Holocarboxylase synthetase deficiency 200
Hookworm infections 89
Human anti-D immunoglobulin 165
Human cytomegalovirus immunoglobulin 165
Human hepatitis B immunoglobulin 166
Human immunodeficiency virus 122
Human papillomovirus
  infection 194
  vaccine 194
Human rabies immunoglobulin 167
Human tetanus immunoglobulin 167
Hydatid disease 88
Hydralazine 100, 201
Hydrochlorothiazide 157
Hydrocortisone 152, 227
Hydrogen sulfide 60
Hydroxycarbamide 212
Hydroxyurea 212
Hydroxyzine 68, 95
Hyoscine butylbromide 132
Hyperbaric oxygen 62
Hyperinsulinemia 177
Hyperkalemia 161
  treatment of 162
Hypermagnesemia 162
Hypertension 97, 100
  treatment of 97

Hypocalcemia 161, 162
  treatment of 174
Hypokalemia 162
Hyponatremia 157
  acute symptomatic 163
Hypoparathyroidism 174
Hypoproteinemia 178
Hypotension 162
  treatment of 188
Hypovolemia 178

I

Ibuprofen 3
Idiopathic arthritis, juvenile 4
Idiopathic hypertrophic subaortic stenosis 101
Idiopathic thrombocytopenic purpura, treatment of 165
Idiopathic urticaria, chronic 93
Idoxuridine 139
Imipenem 26
Imipramine 57
Immunodeficiency syndrome 166
Immunoglobulins 165
Indinavir 125
Indomethacin 3
Infantile spasms 75, 153, 176
Inflammatory disorder 6
Influenza
  A virus infection, treatment of 138
  virus vaccine 194
Initial ventilator settings 230t
Insomnia 75
Inspired oxygen, fraction of 229t
Insulin 213
Intactable epilepsy 167
Interferon alfa 140
Intestinal amebiasis 116
Intra-abdominal infection 115
Intracranial pressure, increased 157

Intractable migraine, severe 67
Intralipid 213
Intramuscular adrenaline 133
Intravenous medication 226*t*
Intubation drugs, rapid sequence 230*t*
Ipratropium 13
Iron 172
Isoniazid 127, 201
Isoprinosine 140
Isoproterenol 222
Ispaghula husk 170
Itraconazole 83
Ivermectin 88, 89

J

Japanese encephalitis 195
Jaundice, neonatal 178
Junctional ectopic tachycardia 20

K

Kanamycin 129
    sulfate 23
Kawasaki disease 166
Keratitis 142
Ketamine 214, 227
Ketoconazole 83
Ketorolac 4
Ketotifen 95
Klebsiella 22, 23, 25-28, 30
    pneumoniae 33

L

Labetalol 100
Lactase enzyme 132
Lactulose 170
Lamivudine 123, 140
Lamotrigine 73

Lansoprazole 135
Laxatives 169
Lead poisoning 61
Legionella 36
Leishmaniasis 117
Lennox-Gastaut syndrome 73
Leprosy 105
Levamisole 89
Levetiracetam 73
Levocetrizine 95
Levofloxacin 44, 105, 129
Levosalbutamol 11
Lidocaine 9, 19, 222
Life-threatening
    hyperkalemia 163
    ventricular arrhythmias 17
Lincomycin 34
Lincosamides 34
Linezolid 50, 129
Liothyronine 190, 191
Liquid paraffin 170
Lisinopril 100
Lithium 58
Loperamide 214
Lopinavir 125
Loratadine 95
Lorazepam 73, 68, 227
Losartan potassium 100
Low cardiac output states, treatment of 143
Lumefantrine 108
Lung disease, chronic 141
Lyme disease 47
Lymphatic filariasis 89

M

Macrolides 34
Magnesium 173
    sulfate 162
Maintenance therapy 13

Malaria
    prevention of 112
    prophylaxis 110
    severe 107
    therapy of 107
    treatment of 107, 110
Mania 120
Manic episodes, acute 58
Mannitol 157
Measles 195
    mumps and rubella 195
    prophylaxis 195
Mebendazole 89
Meclizine 66
Meconium aspiration syndrome 230
Mefenamic acid 4
Mefloquine 110
Megaloblastic anemia 200
Melatonin 119
Meloxicam 4
Meningitis, treatment of 29
Meperidine 8
Meropenem 26, 227
Metabolic acidosis 163, 228
Metabolic alkalosis 228
Methemoglobinemia 60, 62
Methocarbamol 184
Methotrexate 214
Methyl alcohol ingestion 62
Methyldopa 101
Methylene blue 62
Methylphenidate 119
Methylprednisolone 153, 227
Metoclopramide 66, 227
Metolazone 157
Metoprolol 101
Metronidazole 115, 227
Mexiletine 19
Micafungin 83
Miconazole 83
Microcytic hypochromic anemia,
    treatment of 172

Midazolam 74, 227
Migraine prophylaxis 56, 101, 103
Milrinone 144
Minerals 172
Minocycline 46, 105
Minoxidil 101
Mometasone 153
Montelukast 14
Morphine sulfate 7
Motion sickness 66, 93
Moxifloxacin 44, 105, 130
Mucor species 80
Multidrug-resistant
    malaria 108
    tuberculosis, drugs for 128
Mupirocin 50, 215
Muscle weakness 150
Musculoskeletal pain 4
Myalgia 5
Myasthenia gravis 113, 176
Mycobacterium tuberculosis 22
Mycoplasma 27, 46, 48
    disease 47
Myotonia, congenital 19
Myotonic dystrophy 19

N

Nadifloxacin 44
Nalidixic acid 44
Naloxone 63
Naproxen 5
Narcotic analgesic 6
Nausea 66, 67
    treatment of 65
Neisseria 43
Nelfinavir 125
Neomycin 23
Neoplastic disorders 153
Neostigmine 64, 113
Nephrogenic diabetes insipidus 3
Nephrotic syndrome 151, 153, 178

Netilmicin sulfate 24
Neuropathic pain 57
Nevirapine 124
Niacin 201
Niclosamide 90
Nicotinic acid 201
Nifedipine 101
Nimesulide 5
Nitazoxanide 115
Nitrazepam 75
Nitrofurantoin 50
Nitroglycerin 199
Nitroprusside 102, 199
Nocturnal enuresis 56
Non-myeloid malignancies, treatment of 147
Non-narcotic analgesic 1
Non-nucleoside reverse transcriptase inhibitors 124
Nonsteroidal anti-inflammatory drugs, treatment of 135
Non-stimulant drug 118
Norepinephrine 188, 223
Norfloxacin 45
Nortriptyline 58
Nucleoside 122
Nutritional biotin deficiency 200
Nutritional supplement 174, 200
Nystatin 84

O

Obsessive-compulsive disorder 57, 58
Octreotide 63, 177
Ofloxacin 45, 105
Olanzepine 120, 215
Omeprazole 135
Onchocerciasis 89
Ondansetron 67, 227
Oral polio vaccine 196
Oral rehydration solution 215
Ornidazole 116
Oseltamivir 140
Osteoarthritis 2, 3
Osteomalacia 174
Osteoporosis 150
Otitis externa 45
  treatment of 50
Otitis media, acute 32
Oxcarbazepine 75
Oxymetazoline 189
Oxytetracycline 46

P

Pain 4, 5
  management of 8
Palonosetron 67
Pancreatin 215
Pancuronium bromide 215
Panic disorder 58
Pantoprazole 136
Para-aminosalicylic acid 127
Paracetamol 5, 59, 183
Paraldehyde 75
Parenteral nutrition 229*t*
Paromomycin sulfate 116
Paroxysmal atrial tachycardia 19
Paroxysmal supraventricular tachycardia, treatment of 17
Paroxysmal ventricular tachycardia 20
Peak inspiratory pressure 230
Pediculosis 89, 180
Pegfilgrastim 149
Penicillin 37
  G aqueous 40
  G benzathine 40
  G procaine 41
  V potassium 41
Pentamidine 116
Pentazocine 8
Peptic ulcer 150

Permethrin 181
Persistent pulmonary hypertension, treatment of 199
Pertussis 36, 192
Pethidine 8
Pharyngitis 32
Phenazopyridine 10
Pheniramine 96
Phenobarbital 75, 227
Phenothiazine-induced dystonic reactions 61
Phenoxybenzamine 102, 199
Phentolamine 102, 199
Phenylephrine 102, 189, 223
Phenytoin 1976, 227
Pheochromocytoma, treatment of 102
Pholcodine 216
Physostigmine 63
Phytomenadione 64
Pilocarpine 63
Pimozide 120
Pinworms 90
Piperacillin 42, 227
Piperazine 90
Piracetam 216
Piroxicam 6
Pituitary hormones 176
Plasma volume 178
Plasmodium falciparum 108
Pneumococcal vaccine 196
Poisoning 59
Polio vaccine, inactivated 194
Poliomyelitis prophylaxis 194
Polyarticular disease 151
Polyethylene glycol 171
Polymyxin B sulfate 50
Portal hypertension 199
Postanoxic myoclonus 73
Postherpetic neuralgia 9
Post-traumatic stress disorder 58

Potassium 173
  chloride 162
  sparing diuretics 155
Pralidoxime 63
Praziquantel 90
Prazocin 64, 103, 199
Prednisolone 153
Premature ventricular contractions 19
Prematurity, apnea of 11
Primaquine 110
Primidone 77
Probenecid 87
Procainamide 19
Prochlorperazine 67
Promethazine 68, 96
Propafenone hydrochloride 20
Propantheline bromide 132
Prophylaxis 194
Propionic acidemias 200
Propofol 216
Propranolol 20, 103
Propylthiouracil 190
Prostaglandin E1 217
Protamine 64, 160
Protease inhibitors 124
Proteus 22, 23, 25, 28
Prothinamide 130
Proton pump inhibitor 135
Pseudoephedrine 96, 189
Pseudomembranous colitis 34
Pseudomonas 22, 24, 25
  aeruginosa 28
Psoriatic arthritis 2
Psychosis 119
Pulmonary edema 158
Pyrantel pamoate 91
Pyrazinamide 128
Pyridostigmine 114
Pyridoxine 64, 77, 201
  dependent seizures 77
Pyrimethamine 110, 111

Q

Quinidine sulfate 20
Quinine 111
Quinolones 43

R

Rabies 196
    prophylaxis against 196
Racecadotril 217
Ramipril 104
Ranitidine 164, 227
Rectal fissures 9
Red man syndrome 53
Renal failure
    acute 157
    chronic 161
Renal rickets 174
Respiratory acidosis 228
Respiratory alkalosis 228
Respiratory distress syndrome 230
Rh isoimmunization 165
Rheumatic carditis, treatment of 153
Rheumatic fever prophylaxis 40
Rheumatoid arthritis 2-4
Rheumatoid disorder 4-6
Ribavirin 141, 202
Riboflavin deficiency, treatment of 202
Ribonucleic acid 122
Rickets 204
Rickettsia 45
Rifampicin 105, 106, 128
Rifaximin 51
Rimantadine 141
Risperidone 120
Ritonavir 125
Rotavirus gastroenteritis prophylaxis 197
Roundworms 90
Roxithromycin 37
Rubella 197
    infection prophylaxis 197

S

Saccharomyces boulardii 217
Salbutamol 11, 14
Salmeterol 15
Salmonella 43, 4, 49
Salts, values of 228t
Scabicidal agents 180
Scabies 89, 180
Schizophrenia 56, 120, 121
Scorpion bite 64
Seasonal allergic
    conjunctivitis 4
    rhinitis 14
Secnidazole 117
Sedatives 118
Seizures
    management of 72
    treatment of 69
Selenium sulfide 217
Sepsis, treatment of 29
Septic shock 151
Serratia 22, 23, 25
    marcescens 46
Sertaconazole 84
Sertraline 58
Serum concentration monitoring 21
Shigella 23, 43, 49
Shock 199
    treatment of 188
Sildenafil 218
Silver sufadiazine 51
Silymarin 218
Simethicone 218
Sinusitis 5
Sisomycin 24
Skeletal muscle relaxants 182
Skin
    diseases 153
    drug 185
    peeling 185
Snakebite 133

Sodium
  bicarbonate 64, 163
  chloride 163
  cromoglycate 15
  nitrite 60
  nitroprusside 104
  picosulfate 171
  stibogluconate 117
  thiosulfate 60
Soft tissue infection 27
Somatropin 177
Sore throat pain 9
Sotalol 20
Spinal cord lesions spasticity 182
Spironolactone 158
Sports injury 5
Staphylococcus 30, 33
  aureus 25, 34, 50
  haemolyticus 28
  pyogenes 34
Status asthmaticus 152
Status epilepticus 72, 73
Stavudine 123
Stevens-Johnson syndrome 34
Stool softener agents 169
Streptococcus 30
  pharyngitis 34, 40
Streptomycin 24
Stress ulcer, prevention of 136
Strongyloidosis 89
Sucralfate 136
Sucrose solution 219
Sulbactam 39
Sulfadoxine 110
Sulfamethoxazole 52
Sulfonylurea poisoning 63
Sympathomimetics 187
Systemic anaerobic infections 115

T

Tachyarrhythmias, supraventricular 20
Tachycardia, supraventricular 20
Tacrolimus 220
Taenia solium 88
Tapeworm infections, treatment of 90
Tazobactam 42
Teicoplanin 51
Terbinafine 84
Terbutaline 15
Tetanus 192, 198
  antitoxin 134
  diphtheria, pertussis 197
  treatment of 134
Tetracycline 45, 47, 111
Theophylline 16
Thiamine 202
Thiazide diuretics 155
Thiobendazole 91
Thiopental 77
Thioridazine 120
Thromboembolic disorders, treatment of 54
Thrombophlebitis 5
Thyroid agent 190
Thyroidectomy 190
Thyrotoxicosis 190
Thyroxine 191
Tic disorders 120
Ticarcillin 42, 43
Tigecycline 47
Tinea infection 82
Tinidazole 117
Tinocardia 220
Tobramycin 25
Tolazoline 199
Tolnaftate 84
Tonic-clonic serizure 73
Tonsillitis 32
Toothache 9
Topiramate 78
Torsemide 158
Tourette syndrome 119, 120
Toxic shock 152

Tramadol hydrochloride 8
Tranexamic acid 160
Transfusional hemosiderosis 145
Transient redness 185
Trauma, abdominal 165
Traumatic ocular hyphema 159
Traveler's diarrhea 51
Tretinoin 186
Triamcinolone 154
Triamterene 158
Trichinosis 88
Trichuriasis 89
Trichuris trichiura 8
Triclofos 121
Trifluoperazine 68, 121
Trifluridine 142
Trigeminal neuralgia 182
Trimethoprim 52
Typhoid 198

U

Ulcer, chronic 51
Urinary analgesic 10
Urinary fibrinolysis 159
Urinary tract infection 27
Ursodeoxycholic acid 220

V

Valproate sodium 78
Vancomycin 52, 227
Varicella 198
    zoster immunoglobulin 168
Vasopressin 144, 177, 223
Venous blood gases 229*t*
Venous thromboembolism,
    treatment of 54
Ventricular arrhythmias 9, 19, 20
Ventricular tachyarrhythmias 20
Ventricular tachycardia 19
Verapamil 104
Vertigo 66, 67
    treatment of 65

Vigabatrin 79
Viral infection 166
Visceral larva migrans 88
Vitamin 200
    A 136, 203
    B_1 202
    B_{12} 200
    B_2 202
    B_3 201
    B_6 201
    C 203
    D 136, 204
    D deficiency 204
    E 136, 204
    K 64, 136, 205
Vomiting 66, 67
    treatment of 65
Voriconazole 84

W

Warfarin 55
    poisoning 64
Wernicke's encephalopathy 202
West syndrome 176
Wilson's disease 146

X

Xylometazoline 189

Y

Yellow fever 198

Z

Zafirlukast 16
Zanamivir 142
Zidovudine 124
Zileuton 16
Zinc 173
Zonisamide 79
Zosprin tablet 1

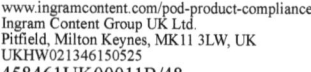

www.ingramcontent.com/pod-product-compliance
Ingram Content Group UK Ltd.
Pitfield, Milton Keynes, MK11 3LW, UK
UKHW021346150525
458461UK00011B/48